# Fluid, Electrolyte, and Acid-Base Balance

D0980421

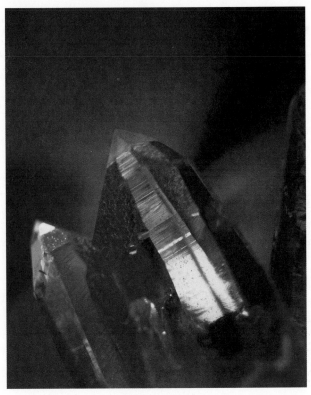

Quartz crystals

## POCKET GUIDE TO

# Fluid, Electrolyte, and Acid-Base Balance

**Ursula Heitz, RN, MSN**
Nursing Consultant
Nashville, Tennessee

**Mima M. Horne, RN, MSN, CDE, BC-ADM**
Staff Nurse
New Hanover Regional Medical Center
Adjunct Faculty
University of North Carolina at Wilmington
Wilmington, North Carolina

*With contributions by*

**Deborah L. Spahn, RD, CNSD**
Registered Dietitian, Metabolic Support Services
Baptist Hospital
Nashville, Tennessee

**FIFTH EDITION**

ELSEVIER
MOSBY

# ELSEVIER
# MOSBY

11830 Westline Industrial Drive
St. Louis, Missouri 63146

POCKET GUIDE TO FLUID, ELECTROLYTE, AND ACID-BASE BALANCE,
FIFTH EDITION                                    ISBN: 0-323-02603-6
Copyright © 2005, 2001, 1997, 1993, 1989 by Mosby Inc.

---

## Notice

Nursing is an ever-changing field. Standard safety precautions must be followed,
but as new research and clinical experience broaden our knowledge, changes in
treatment and drug therapy may become necessary or appropriate. Readers are
advised to check the most current product information provided by the manufacturer of each drug to be administered to verify the recommended dose, the method
and duration of administration, and contraindications. It is the responsibility of the
licensed prescriber, relying on experience and knowledge of the patient, to determine
dosages and the best treatment for each individual patient. Neither the publisher nor
the author assumes any liability for any injury and/or damage to persons or property
arising from this publication.

The Publisher.

---

Previous editions copyrighted 1989, 1993, 1997, 2001.

*Executive Editor:* Michael S. Ledbetter
*Senior Developmental Editor:* Laurie K. Gower
*Publishing Services Manager:* Patricia Tannian
*Senior Project Manager:* Anne Altepeter
*Book Design Manager:* Gail Morey Hudson

Printed in China

**Library of Congress Cataloging-in-Publication Data**

Heitz, Ursula.
    Pocket guide to fluid, electrolyte, and acid-base balance/Ursula Heitz,
Mima M. Horne; with contributions by Deborah L. Spahn. – 5th ed.
        p.cm.
    Includes bibliographical references and index.
    ISBN 0-323-02603-6
1. Body fluid disorders–Nursing–Handbooks, manuals, etc. 2. Water-electrolyte
imbalances–Nursing–Handbooks, manuals, etc. I. Horne, Mima M. II. Spahn,
Deborah L. III. Title.
RC630.P63 2005
616.3'992–dc22                                                    2004050683

Last digit is the print number:  9  8  7  6  5  4  3  2  1

# Preface

*Pocket Guide to Fluid, Electrolyte, and Acid-Base Balance,* fifth edition, was developed to provide nursing students and practicing nurses with quick, practical information about pathophysiology, assessment, diagnostic tests, collaborative management, nursing diagnoses, and nursing interventions for patients with fluid, electrolyte, and acid-base imbalances. The book is distinctive in that, despite its portable size, its coverage of content is both extensive and concise. The organization of the fourth edition has been retained, including the use of unit subdivisions to facilitate retrieval of content. Each disorder is presented in a consistent format to enhance utility in the clinical environment. The outline format, boldface headings, use of color, and illustrations reinforce the book's clarity and further enhance its usability. The inclusion of numerous tables and charts allows for quick review of information. In addition, all efforts have been made to ensure that the level of presentation is as easy to understand as possible.

Nurses can use this reference for three purposes:

1. To review basic physiologic concepts regarding fluid, electrolyte, and acid-base balance. This concise review assists in application of the content presented in Units II and III.
2. To identify a patient's specific fluid, electrolyte, or acid-base disturbance (discussed in Unit II) and review the nursing diagnoses and care for that specific disturbance.
3. To identify the medical diagnoses (e.g., diabetic ketoacidosis) (in Unit III) and review the list of fluid, electrolyte, and acid-base disturbances associated with that particular disorder (e.g., hypokalemia, hypovolemia, metabolic acidosis), and then refer to the chapters in Unit II that cover these disturbances in detail.

This edition has been thoroughly revised and updated, with the addition of content that is relevant for the whole spectrum of patient care and that is as applicable to critical care as to the subacute setting (home care). Whenever possible, content related to pediatric and geriatric patients has been expanded. Although this fifth edition includes more detailed information about infants and children, the reader is advised that all specific numbers refer to adults unless otherwise noted. As before, the appendices are unusually detailed. The appendices include standard abbreviations, a glossary of terms, and normal values for laboratory tests discussed in the text, as well as tables describing the effects of age on fluid, electrolyte, and acid-base balance.

Updates on new medications and interventions for treating electrolyte imbalances are also included. A new, more complete, and easy-to-reference chart combines the causes and classification of metabolic acidosis. This edition provides an updated and reorganized chart on etiologies of acute pancreatitis, with clearly identified subsets. Also included is new information on current research and application of that research to the clinical setting regarding patients with adult respiratory distress syndrome. Clinical guidelines are included.

Standard abbreviations are used in this text. We encourage readers to follow hospital or agency guidelines when documenting in patient charts and communicating with other health care professionals in a written format.

We wish to thank our contributor, Deborah L. Spahn, for a job well done. We appreciate the expertise she brought to her chapter on nutritional support. The chapter has been revised, with the addition of a clear and concise table outlining types of enteral formulations.

*Pocket Guide to Fluid, Electrolyte, and Acid-Base Balance* was written to supplement medical-surgical textbooks and assumes the reader has a basic understanding of physiology, pathophysiology, and assessment. The book also serves as a resource for practicing nurses and academicians. The primary goals are to make information about fluids, electrolytes, acid-base balance, and related topics understandable and to facilitate application of that information to patient care. Reviewers indicate that these objectives have been achieved, and comments and suggestions from our readers are welcome, so that we may enhance the book's usefulness in future editions.

Ursula Heitz
Mima M. Horne

# Contents

# BASIC
# PRINCIPLES

I

# Overview of Fluid and Electrolyte Balance

1

The cell is the fundamental functioning unit of the human body. For cells to perform their individual physiologic tasks, a stable environment is necessary, including maintenance of a steady supply of nutrients and continuous removal of metabolic wastes. Careful regulation of body fluids helps ensure a stable internal environment.

## Composition of Body Fluids

All body fluids are dilute solutions of water and dissolved substances (solutes).

### Water

Water is the major constituent of the human body. The average adult male is approximately 60% water by weight; the average female is approximately 50% to 55% water. Factors that affect body water include:

1. **Fat cells:** These contain little water; thus body water decreases with increasing body fat.
2. **Age:** As a rule, body water decreases with increasing age. Premature infants may be as much as 80% water by weight, whereas a full-term infant is approximately 70% water. By the age of 6 months to 1 year, body water decreases to approximately 60%, with little further reduction throughout childhood. An older adult may be 45% to 55% water by weight because of an increase in body fat. The percentage of water also decreases in older adults as muscle mass declines (Table 1-1).

Table 1-1    Changes in total body water with age

| Age | Kilogram Weight (%) |
| --- | --- |
| Premature infant | 80 |
| 3 months | 70 |
| 6 months | 60 |
| 1-2 years | 59 |
| 11-16 years | 58 |
| Adult | 58-60 |
| Obese adult | 40-50 |
| Emaciated adult | 70-75 |

From Groer MW: *Physiology and pathophysiology of the body fluids,* St Louis, 1981, Mosby.

3. **Female gender:** Women have proportionately less body water because of proportionately greater body fat.

## Solutes

In addition to water, body fluids contain two types of dissolved substances (solutes): electrolytes and nonelectrolytes.

1. **Electrolytes:** Substances that dissociate (separate) in solution and conduct an electric current. Electrolytes dissociate into positive and negative ions and are measured by their capacity to combine with each other (milliequivalents/liter [mEq/L]), by their molecular weight in grams (millimoles/liter [mmol/L]), or by weight (milligrams/deciliter [mg/dL]). The number of cations and anions in solution, as measured in milliequivalents, is always equal.

   ■ *Cations:* Ions that develop a positive charge in solution. The primary extracellular cation is sodium ($Na^+$), whereas the primary intracellular cation is potassium ($K^+$). A pump system exists in the wall of body cells and pumps out sodium and in potassium.

   ■ *Anions:* Ions that develop a negative charge in solution. The primary extracellular anions are chloride ($Cl^-$) and bicarbonate ($HCO_3^-$), whereas the primary intracellular anion is phosphate ion ($PO_4^{3-}$).

   Because the electrolyte content of the plasma and interstitial fluid (ISF) is essentially the same (Table 1-2), plasma electrolyte values reflect the composition of the extracellular

Table 1-2  Primary constituents of body fluid compartments

| Compartment | Na⁺ (mmol/L) | K⁺ (mmol/L) | Cl⁻ (mmol/L) | HCO₃⁻ (mmol/L) | PO₄³⁻ (mEq/L) |
|---|---|---|---|---|---|
| Intravascular (plasma) | 142 | 4.5 | 104 | 24 | 2.0 |
| Interstitial | 145 | 4.4 | 117 | 27 | 2.3 |
| Intracellular (skeletal muscle cell) | 12 | 150.0 | 4 | 12 | 40.0 |
| Transcellular |  |  |  |  |  |
| Gastric juice | 60 | 7.0 | 100 | 0 | — |
| Pancreatic juice | 130 | 7.0 | 60 | 100 | — |
| Sweat | 45 | 5.0 | 58 | 0 | — |

This is a partial list. Other constituents include calcium ion ($Ca^{2+}$), magnesium ion ($Mg^{2+}$), sulfates, proteinates, and organic acids.

NOTE: Average values are given.

Modified from Rose BD: *Clinical physiology of acid-base and electrolyte disorders*, ed 3, New York, 1989, McGraw-Hill.

fluid (ECF), which is composed of intravascular fluid (IVF) and ISF (see the section on Fluid Compartments). However, plasma electrolyte values do not necessarily reflect the electrolyte composition of the intracellular fluid (ICF). Understanding the difference between these two compartments is important in anticipating the types of imbalances that can occur with certain disorders such as tissue trauma or acid-base imbalances. In these situations, electrolytes may be released from or move into or out of the cells, significantly altering plasma electrolyte values (see the discussions of potassium balance, Chapter 8, and phosphorus balance, Chapter 10). Regulation of individual electrolyte levels is critical to the maintenance of body fluid osmolality, acid-base balance, neuromuscular function, and cellular metabolism.

2. **Nonelectrolytes:** Substances such as glucose and urea that do not dissociate in solution and are measured by weight (milligrams per 100 mL [deciliter], or mg/dL). Other clinically important nonelectrolytes include creatinine and bilirubin.

# Fluid Compartments

Body fluids are distributed between two major fluid compartments: the intracellular compartment and the extracellular compartment (Figure 1-1).

## Intracellular Fluid

Intracellular fluid is the fluid contained within the cells. In adults, approximately two thirds of the body's fluid is intracellular; this is approximately 27 L in the average (70-kilogram [kg]) adult male. In contrast, only half of an infant's body fluid is intracellular.

## Extracellular Fluid

Extracellular fluid is the fluid outside the cells. The relative size of ECF decreases with advancing age. In the newborn, approximately half the body fluid is contained within ECF. After 1 year of age, the relative volume of ECF decreases to approximately one third of the total volume. This equals approximately 15 L in the average (70-kg) adult male. ECF is

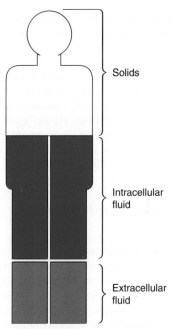

Figure 1-1
Comparison of intracellular fluid with extracellular fluid.

further divided into the following:

1. **Interstitial fluid:** Fluid surrounding the cells, equal to approximately 11 to 12 L in adults. Lymph fluid is included in the interstitial volume. Relative to body size, the volume of ISF is approximately twice as great in the newborn as in the adult.

2. **Intravascular fluid:** Fluid contained within the blood vessels (i.e., the plasma volume). The relative volume of IVF is similar in adults and children. Average adult blood volume is approximately 5 to 6 L, of which about 3 L is plasma. The remaining 2 to 3 L consist of red blood cells (RBCs, or erythrocytes), which transport oxygen and act as important body buffers; white blood cells (WBCs, or leukocytes); and platelets. Functions of the blood include:

   ▪ Delivery of nutrients (e.g., glucose, oxygen) to the tissues

- Transport of waste products to the kidneys and lungs
- Delivery of antibodies and WBCs to sites of infection
- Transport of hormones to their sites of action
- Circulation of body heat

3. **Transcellular fluid (TCF):** Fluid contained within specialized cavities of the body. Examples of TCF include cerebrospinal, pericardial, pleural, synovial, and intraocular fluids, and digestive secretions. At any given time, TCF is approximately 1 L. However, large amounts of fluid may move into and out of the transcellular space each day. For example, the gastrointestinal (GI) tract normally secretes and reabsorbs up to 3 to 6 L per day.

# Factors That Affect Movement of Water and Solutes
## Membranes

Each of the fluid compartments is separated by a selectively permeable membrane that permits the movement of water and some solutes. Although small molecules such as urea and water move freely among all compartments, certain substances move less readily. Plasma proteins, for example, are restricted to the IVF because of the low permeability of the capillary membrane to large molecules. Selective permeability of membranes helps maintain the unique composition of each compartment while allowing for movement of nutrients from the plasma to the cells and movement of waste products out of the cells and (eventually) into the plasma. The body's semipermeable membranes include:

1. **Cell membranes:** Separate ICF from ISF and are composed of lipids and protein.
2. **Capillary membranes:** Separate IVF from ISF.
3. **Epithelial membranes:** Separate ISF and IVF from TCF. Examples of epithelial membranes include the mucosal epithelium of the stomach and intestines, the synovial membrane, and the renal tubules.

## Transport Processes

In addition to membrane selectivity, the movement of water and solutes is determined by several transport processes (Figure 1-2).

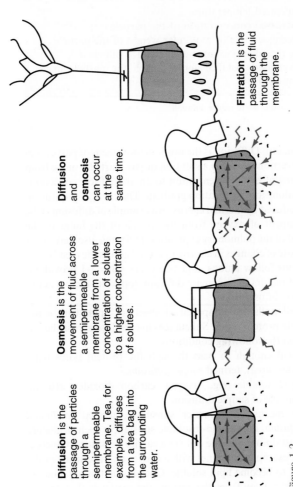

**Diffusion** is the passage of particles through a semipermeable membrane. Tea, for example, diffuses from a tea bag into the surrounding water.

**Osmosis** is the movement of fluid across a semipermeable membrane from a lower concentration of solutes to a higher concentration of solutes.

**Diffusion** and **osmosis** can occur at the same time.

**Filtration** is the passage of fluid through the membrane.

Figure 1-2
**Transport processes.**
(Modified from Oberley ET et al: *Core curriculum for dialysis technicians: module 1: today's dialysis environment: an overview,* 1992, Medical Media Publishing.)

---

## Box 1-1    Factors That Increase Diffusion*

- Increased temperature
- Increased concentration of the particle
- Decreased size or molecular weight of the particle
- Increased surface area available for diffusion
- Decreased distance across which the particle mass must diffuse

---

*Opposite factors act to reduce diffusion.

1. **Diffusion:** Diffusion is the random movement of particles in all directions through a solution or gas. Particles move from an area of high concentration to an area of low concentration along a concentration gradient. The energy for diffusion is produced by thermal energy. An example of diffusion is the movement of oxygen from the alveoli of the lungs to the blood of the pulmonary capillaries. Diffusion also may occur because of changes in electric potential across the membrane. Cations follow anions, and vice versa. (Box 1-1 provides a list of factors that increase diffusion [opposite factors act to reduce diffusion].)

    Cell walls are composed of sheets of lipids with many minute protein pores. Substances may diffuse across the cell wall in the following conditions:
    - Small enough to pass through the protein pores (e.g., water, urea), termed *simple diffusion.*
    - Lipid soluble (e.g., oxygen, carbon dioxide), also an example of simple diffusion.
    - By means of a carrier substance, termed *facilitated diffusion.* Large lipid-insoluble substances such as glucose must diffuse into the cell via a carrier substance. Glucose, for example, combines with a carrier on the outside of the cell to become lipid soluble. Once inside the cell, glucose breaks away from the carrier; the carrier is then free to facilitate diffusion of additional glucose.

    As with simple diffusion, facilitated diffusion requires the presence of a concentration gradient that favors diffusion. The rate of facilitated diffusion, however, depends on the availability of the carrier substance. With a large concentration gradient (i.e., the difference between the areas of high and low concentration is great), the carrier can become saturated (used up) and diffusion decreases despite the presence of a favorable concentration gradient. Glucose moves into the cell, for example, only with a favorable concentration gradient and an available carrier substance.

2. **Active transport:** Simple diffusion does not occur in the absence of a favorable electric or concentration gradient. Energy is required for a substance to move from an area of lesser or equal concentration to an area of equal or higher concentration. This is termed *active transport,* and like facilitated diffusion, it depends on the availability of carrier substances. Many important solutes are transported actively across cell membranes and include sodium, potassium, hydrogen, glucose, and amino acids. The renal tubules, for example, depend on active transport to reabsorb all the glucose filtered by the glomeruli, which allows excretion of glucose-free urine. As with facilitated diffusion, the carriers can become overwhelmed or saturated. In the case of glucose within the renal tubule, saturation occurs when the blood glucose exceeds approximately 180 to 200 mg/dL. Active transport is vital for maintaining the unique composition of both the ECF and the ICF.

3. **Filtration:** Filtration is the movement of water and solutes from an area of high hydrostatic pressure to an area of low hydrostatic pressure. Hydrostatic pressure is the pressure created by the weight of fluid. Filtration is important in directing fluid from the arterial end of the capillaries and is also the force that enables the kidneys to filter 180 L of plasma a day.

4. **Osmosis:** Osmosis is the movement of water across a semipermeable membrane from an area of lower solute concentration to an area of higher solute concentration. Osmosis can occur across any membrane when the solute concentrations on either side of the membrane change. The following terms are associated with osmosis:

   - *Osmotic pressure:* The amount of hydrostatic pressure necessary to stop the osmotic flow of water.
   - *Oncotic pressure:* The osmotic pressure exerted by colloids (proteins). Albumin, for example, exerts oncotic pressure

within the blood vessels and helps hold the water content of the blood in the intravascular space (IVS).

■ *Osmotic diuresis:* Increased urine output caused by substances such as mannitol, glucose, or contrast media, which are excreted in the urine and reduce renal water resorption. For example, an osmotic diuresis occurs in uncontrolled diabetes mellitus because of excess glucose in the renal tubule. When the blood glucose is within normal range, all the glucose filtered by the kidney is reabsorbed (saved) via active transport. In hyperglycemia (blood glucose level >180 to 200 mg/dL), the kidneys' ability to reabsorb glucose is overwhelmed (i.e., the carrier substance becomes saturated). The glucose that is not reabsorbed remains in the tubule and acts osmotically to hold water that otherwise would be reabsorbed. The net result is glucosuria and polyuria.

## Concentration of Body Fluids

1. **Osmolality:** As discussed previously, changes in the concentration of body fluids affect the movement of water among fluid compartments by osmosis. The measure of a solution's ability to create osmotic pressure and thus affect the movement of water is termed *osmolality.* Osmolality also may be described as a measure of the concentration of body fluids (the ratio of solutes to water) because it is reported in milliosmoles per kilogram (mOsm/kg) of water. One osmole contains $6 \times 10^{23}$ particles. *Osmolarity,* another term used to describe the concentration of solutions, reflects the number of particles in a liter of solution and is measured in mOsm/L. Because body fluids are relatively dilute, the difference between osmolality and osmolarity is small and the terms often are used interchangeably. Osmolality is the measure used to evaluate serum and urine in clinical practice.

Changes in extracellular osmolality may result in changes in both ECF and ICF volume:

*Decreased ECF osmolality → movement of water from the ECF to the ICF*

*Increased ECF osmolality → movement of water from the ICF to the ECF*

Water continues to move until the osmolality of the two compartments reaches equilibrium. This is the rationale for the use of intravenous mannitol in the treatment of cerebral edema. Mannitol increases the osmolality of the ECF, promoting the movement of water out of the cerebral cells and thereby reducing cellular swelling.

Osmolality of the ECF may be determined with measuring serum osmolality (see Chapter 5). Sodium is the primary determinant of ECF osmolality. Because sodium is limited primarily to the ECF, it acts to hold water in that compartment. Potassium helps maintain the volume of ICF, and the plasma proteins help maintain the volume of the IVS.

2. **Tonicity:** Small molecules like urea and alcohol that readily cross all membranes quickly equilibrate among compartments and have little effect on the movement of water. These small molecules are termed *ineffective osmoles*. In contrast, sodium, glucose, and mannitol are examples of *effective osmoles;* they do not cross the cell membrane quickly and therefore affect the movement of water. Thus *effective osmolality* (i.e., osmolality that causes water to move from one compartment to another) is dependent not only on the number of solutes but also on the permeability of the membrane to these solutes. *Tonicity* is another term for effective osmolality.

   ■ *Isotonic solutions:* Solutions with the same effective osmolality as body fluids (approximately 280 to 300 mOsm/kg). An example is normal saline solution—0.9% sodium chloride (NaCl) solution.

   ■ *Hypotonic solutions:* Solutions with an effective osmolality less than that of body fluids. An example is 0.45% NaCl solution.

   ■ *Hypertonic solutions:* Solutions having an effective osmolality greater than that of body fluids. An example is 3% NaCl solution.

   *Clinical hypotonicity* occurs with an abnormal gain in water or a loss of sodium-rich fluids with replacement by water only. *Clinical hypertonicity* may develop because of loss of water (e.g., diabetes insipidus), loss of hypotonic body fluids (e.g., sweating, diarrhea), or gain of effective

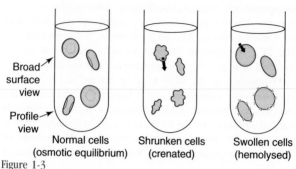

Isotonic solution    Hypertonic solution  Hypotonic solution

Broad
surface
view

Profile
view

Normal cells        Shrunken cells       Swollen cells
(osmotic equilibrium)  (crenated)         (hemolysed)

Figure 1-3
Effect of osmotic pressure on cells.

osmoles (e.g., hyperglycemia; administration of hypertonic
NaCl, sodium bicarbonate, or mannitol). Hyperosmolality
without hypertonicity (which does not cause cellular dehydration) occurs with the ingestion of methyl alcohol or
ethylene glycol or in renal failure from retention of urea.
(Figure 1-3 provides a depiction of osmotic pressure on
the cells.)

# Regulation of Vascular Volume and Extracellular Fluid Osmolality

2

For an optimal environment for the body's cells, the composition, concentration, and volume of the extracellular fluid (ECF) are regulated by a combination of renal, metabolic, and neurologic functions. The ECF is continuously altered and then modified as the body reacts with the external environment. In contrast, the intracellular fluid (ICF) is protected by the ECF and remains relatively stable, ensuring normal cellular function. Because the primary constituents of the ECF are water and sodium (and sodium's accompanying anions), their regulation is crucial for maintenance of the volume and concentration of the ECF (Figures 2-1 to 2-3).

The *total content* of sodium in the ECF determines the ECF volume. If the sodium content of the ECF increases, so does the ECF volume. In contrast, the *concentration* of sodium in the ECF indicates the relative water content of the ECF and whether water moves into or out of the ICF. Decreased concentration of sodium in the ECF (i.e., hyponatremia), for example, indicates a relative increase in ECF water and a movement of water into the ICF. Thus changes in the sodium concentration of the ECF cause changes in the ICF volume.

Regulation of the composition of ECF depends on the regulation of the individual electrolytes (see Chapters 7 through 11).

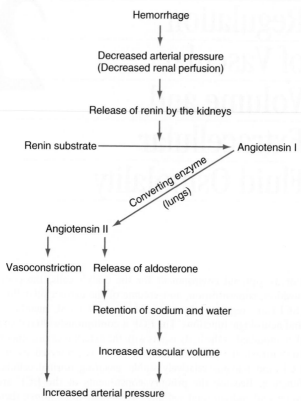

Figure 2-1
Action of renin-angiotensin-aldosterone system: clinical example.

## Regulation of Vascular Volume

Large fluctuations can occur in the volume of the interstitial portion of the ECF without markedly affecting body functions. This is especially true if the changes occur slowly. Individuals with cirrhosis, for example, are often able to tolerate significant amounts of ascitic fluid. The vascular portion of the ECF is less tolerant of change and must be maintained carefully to ensure that the tissues receive an adequate supply of nutrients and

[Vasotec]) act in part by preventing the conversion of angiotensin I to angiotensin II. Another class of antihypertensive medications acts by blocking the angiotensin II tissue receptor (i.e., angiotensin-receptor blockers [ARBs], such as eprosartan [Teveten]). Because these medications decrease the level of angiotensin II, they also reduce the production of aldosterone.

Other actions of angiotensin II include stimulation of thirst and increased absorption of bicarbonate by the renal tubule.

## Aldosterone

Aldosterone is a mineralocorticoid hormone released by the adrenal cortex that acts on the distal portion of the renal tubule to increase the resorption (saving) of sodium and the secretion and excretion of potassium and hydrogen. Because sodium retention leads to water retention, aldosterone acts as an important volume regulator. Factors that increase the release of aldosterone include:

1. Increased angiotensin II levels
2. Increased plasma potassium levels
3. Markedly decreased plasma sodium levels
4. Increased adrenocorticotropic hormone levels

## Natriuretic Peptides

Natriuretic peptides are a family of peptide hormones that affect fluid volume status and cardiovascular function through increased excretion of sodium (natriuresis), direct vasodilation, and opposition of the renin-angiotensin-aldosterone system. Three separate peptides have been identified: A-type produced by the atrial myocardium, B-type produced by the ventricular myocardium, and C-type produced by the vascular endothelium. A-type and B-type peptides are released in response to increased pressure within the heart, and C-type peptides are released in response to vascular shear stress (see Fig 2-3). Increased levels of natriuretic peptides occur in any condition that causes volume expansion or elevated cardiac pressures (e.g., congestive heart failure [CHF], chronic renal failure, use of vasoconstrictor agents, and atrial tachycardia).

As *analogs* (manmade substances with similar structure and function) of the natriuretic peptide hormones are developed, they may be useful in the management of hypertension, CHF, renal failure, and other volume overload states. Currently, a recombinant form of B-type natriuretic peptide, nesiritide (Natrecor), is used in the treatment of acute decompensated CHF. Point of care measurement of the B-type natriuretic peptide level (BNP) is now used to assist in the diagnosis and classification of CHF.

## Antidiuretic Hormone and Thirst

Both antidiuretic hormone (ADH) and thirst assist in the regulation of vascular volume. (See the subsequent sections for a discussion of their actions.)

# Regulation of Extracellular Fluid Osmolality

Because the number of particles within most cells remains relatively constant and cell membranes are permeable to water, changes in the concentration of the fluid surrounding the cells affect the volume of water within the cells. Thus the concentration or osmolality of the ECF determines whether fluid moves into or out of the cells.

*Increased ECF osmolality → cells shrivel*
*Decreased ECF osmolality → cells swell*

Thus it is critical that the ECF osmolality be maintained within a narrow range to protect cellular function and the volume of the ICF. The primary symptoms of altered plasma osmolality are neurologic (e.g., irritability, personality changes, seizures, coma) and reflect changes in brain-cell function.

Because sodium is the primary solute of the ECF, it is also the primary determinant of ECF osmolality. Two control systems work together to maintain the sodium/water ratio: ADH and thirst.

## Antidiuretic Hormone

Antidiuretic hormone is produced by the hypothalamus and secreted into the general circulation by the posterior pituitary gland. It acts on the collecting duct in the kidney to increase the resorption (saving) of water and to allow the excretion of concentrated urine. ADH is also an arterial vasoconstrictor that acts to raise blood pressure by increasing vascular resistance. ADH is regulated primarily by changes in plasma osmolality and ECV. Additional factors that affect the release of ADH are stress, surgery, and certain medications. (Factors that increase the release of ADH are found in Box 2-1; factors that decrease the release of ADH are found in Box 2-2. See Chapter 20 for a discussion of disorders of ADH.) Because ADH affects the resorption of water only, changes in the release of ADH affect the concentration of sodium in the plasma. For example, increased release of ADH results in a decrease in the plasma sodium level from the retention of increased water. (See Chapter 7 for further discussion of the role of ADH in the regulation of plasma sodium.)

In addition to medications that affect the release of ADH, medications also exist that suppress or enhance the action of ADH on the renal collecting duct (Box 2-3).

---

### Box 2-1    Factors That Increase the Release of Antidiuretic Hormone*

- Increased plasma osmolality sensed by osmoreceptors located within the hypothalamus
- Decreased ECV sensed by volume receptors located within the pulmonary vasculature and left atria
- Decreased blood pressure sensed by baroreceptors
- Stress and pain
- Medications, including morphine and barbiturates
- Surgery and certain anesthetics
- Positive-pressure ventilators

*See Chapter 20 for a discussion of disorders that lead to inappropriate or excessive production of ADH.

---

### Box 2-2    Factors That Decrease the Release of Antidiuretic Hormone*

- Decreased plasma osmolality
- Increased ECV
- Increased blood pressure
- Medications, including phenytoin and ethyl alcohol

*See Chapter 20 for a discussion of disorders that lead to a reduction in ADH activity or release.

> ## Box 2-3  Medications That Alter the Action of Antidiuretic Hormone
>
> **Suppressors**
> - Lithium
> - Demeclocycline
> - Methoxyflurane
>
> **Enhancers**
> - Chlorpropamide
> - Indomethacin

## Thirst

In addition to ADH, thirst also acts to regulate the ECF concentration and is stimulated by essentially the same factors that increase the release of ADH: increased plasma osmolality, volume depletion, and hypotension. Increased angiotensin II levels and dry mucous membranes (the sensation of a dry mouth) also stimulate thirst. Thirst is not as carefully regulated as ADH, as evidenced by the fact that it is affected strongly by social and behavioral factors. In healthy conditions, the amount and timing of fluid intake have more to do with food intake than physiologic regulation. However, thirst does provide the primary protection against hyperosmolality during illness or stress. Symptomatic hyperosmolality occurs only in individuals who do not have a normal thirst mechanism or who do not have access to adequate water. Thus hyperosmolality typically occurs in infants or comatose patients who are unable to ask for water. Alert patients with diabetes insipidus, for example, who excrete a large, abnormally dilute urine because of altered ADH function, maintain a relatively normal osmolality and volume as long as they are able to drink and satisfy their thirst.

## Defense of Brain Cell Volume

Although affected by changes in ECF osmolality, especially sudden changes, the brain cells are uniquely able to defend against large changes in water volume by varying the number of intracellular particles. This is an important defense, given the critical function and location of the brain. The exact particles involved and the mechanism by which these changes occur remain unclear. Rapid correction of abnormalities in ECF osmolality (e.g., rapid correction of hyponatremia, hypernatremia, or extreme hyperglycemia) must be avoided because of the risk of sudden and symptomatic changes in brain cell volume (see Chapter 7).

# Fluid Gains and Losses

3

In periods of health, a steady state, or balance, exists between the fluids gained and lost by the body. As discussed in Chapter 2, the volume, concentration, and composition of body fluids are regulated so that output matches intake and balance is maintained. Loss of hypotonic fluids, for example, leads to decreased water excretion and increased thirst. The body's physiologic balance is termed *homeostasis*. This chapter reviews the means of normal and abnormal fluid gains and losses. (Table 3-1 lists daily fluid gains and losses in approximate amounts.) Unless otherwise specified, all volumes refer to those in the healthy adult.

## Fluid Gains
### Oxidative Metabolism

Approximately 250 to 300 milliliters (mL) of water are produced daily with the oxidation of carbohydrates, proteins, and fat. That is, oxygen combines with some of the hydrogen in these substances to produce water. This amount of water is insufficient to compensate for the body's obligatory fluid losses; thus some additional oral, parenteral, or enteral intake is necessary to maintain body volume. In the best conditions, individuals may survive weeks without the intake of food but only days without the intake of water.

### Oral Fluids

In the average adult, approximately 1100 to 1400 mL of fluid are consumed orally per day. Fluid intake varies greatly because thirst is affected by social and behavioral factors and by physiologic factors (see Chapter 2). When a variety of fluids are available, the volume of oral fluid intake typically exceeds the amount necessary to maintain fluid balance.

Table 3-1  Average daily fluid gains and losses in adults

| Fluid Gains | | Fluid Losses | |
|---|---|---|---|
| Oxidative metabolism | 300 mL | Kidneys | 1200-1500 mL |
| | | Skin | 500-600 mL |
| Oral fluids | 1100-1400 mL | Lungs | 400 mL |
| Solid foods | 800-1000 mL | GI tract | 100-200 mL |
| Total | 2200-2700 mL | Total | 2200-2700 mL |

## Solid Food

Fluid is gained through the consumption of solid food, which provides approximately 800 to 1000 mL of water each day. Meat, for example, is approximately 70% water by weight, and fruits and vegetables are more than 90% water.

## Fluid Therapy

Fluid also may be gained through parenteral or enteral routes and with irrigants that are retained. If a nasogastric (NG) tube is irrigated, for example, and an equal amount is not withdrawn and discarded, the extra irrigant must be considered a fluid gain. Mechanical ventilation with humidified gases may result in a net gain of water by the lungs. (See Chapter 6 for a discussion of parenteral fluid therapy and Chapter 26 for a discussion of all types of nutritional therapy.)

# Fluid Losses

## Kidneys

The kidneys are the primary regulators of fluid and electrolyte balance. Approximately 180 liters (L) of plasma are filtered daily by the kidneys of the healthy adult. From this volume, approximately 1500 mL of urine are excreted each day. The volume, composition, and concentration of urine vary greatly and depend on fluid intake and other means of fluid loss. Urine values (volume and concentration) should always be evaluated in relation to the body's need to conserve or excrete fluid. The dehydrated individual who needs to conserve fluid, for example, is expected to excrete less urine than the individual who is adequately hydrated.

The concentration of urine may range from 50 to 1200 milliosmoles (mOsm)/kilogram (kg), although it more typically ranges between 300 and 900 mOsm/kg. Although sodium is the primary determinant of extracellular fluid (ECF) osmolality or concentration, metabolic wastes are the primary determinant of urinary osmolality or concentration. Therefore in severe hypovolemia or hypotension, for example, the kidneys are able to excrete concentrated, yet relatively sodium-free, urine.

1. **Normal urinary output:** At maximal urinary concentration (1200 mOsm/kg), at least 400 mL of urine must be produced to excrete the daily load of metabolic wastes in the adult. Infants, older adults, and individuals with renal disease whose urine cannot be maximally concentrated have greater obligatory water losses; they need to produce a proportionately larger volume of urine to excrete the daily load of metabolic wastes. Average daily urine output is 1500 mL in adults. Hourly urine output has an average range of 40 to 80 mL for adults and 0.5 mL/kg for children.

2. **Oliguria:** Urinary output of less than 400 mL in 24 hours. It signals the retention of metabolic wastes.

3. **Anuria:** Production of less than 100 mL of urine in 24 hours.

4. **Polyuria:** An abnormally large amount of urinary output.

## Skin

An average of 500 to 600 mL of sensible and insensible fluid is lost via the skin each day.

1. **Insensible fluid:** Loss is evaporative from the skin and occurs without the individual's awareness. Fluid is lost at a rate of 6 mL/kg/24 hours in the average adult, but this rate can increase significantly with fever or burns. An adult will lose an additional 100 to 150 mL of fluid daily for each one degree body temperature over 37° C. Infants with a low birth weight, especially those weighing less than 1 kg, are prone to extremely high rates of insensible fluid loss because of multiple factors, including larger relative skin surface area and increased water content in the skin. Use of radiant warmers significantly increases insensible fluid loss in neonates. Insensible fluid is nearly free of electrolytes and should be considered pure water loss.

2. **Sensible fluid (e.g., sweat):** Important in dissipating body heat and, like insensible fluid, hypotonic. Sensible fluid, however, does contain a significant amount of electrolytes (see Table 1-2). The rate of sensible fluid loss varies greatly with the individual's activity level and the ambient temperature. In extreme cases, sensible fluid loss may be as great as 2 L/hour.

## Lungs

Approximately 400 mL of insensible fluid are lost through the lungs each day. This amount may increase with increased respiratory depth or dry climate.

## Gastrointestinal Tract

In normal conditions, the gastrointestinal (GI) tract accounts for only 100 to 200 mL of fluid loss each day, yet it plays a vital role in fluid regulation because it is the site of nearly all fluid gain. In disease, however, the GI tract may become a site of major fluid loss because approximately 3 to 6 L of isotonic fluid are secreted into and reabsorbed out of the GI tract daily. This amount is equal to approximately one third of the ECF volume. Thus abnormal GI losses (e.g., NG suction, vomiting, diarrhea) may lead to profound fluid loss. The composition of the GI secretions varies with the location within the GI tract. Above the pylorus, the losses are isotonic and contain sodium, potassium, chloride, and hydrogen. Below the pylorus, losses are isotonic and contain sodium, potassium, and bicarbonate (see Table 1-2). Diarrhea from the large intestine is hypotonic (see Chapter 18).

## Additional Losses

Significant amounts of fluid may be lost as a result of increased evaporative loss from large open wounds, draining wounds, fistulas, or external bleeding. Crying may contribute significantly to fluid loss in small children.

## Third-Space Losses

The loss of ECF into a normally nonequilibrating space is termed *third-space fluid shift*. Although this fluid is not lost from the body, it is temporarily unavailable for use by either the intracellular fluid (ICF) or ECF. Third-space fluid losses must be considered in evaluation of the adequacy of fluid therapy (see Table 6-1 for a list of disorders associated with third-space fluid shifts). A patient with a significant third-space fluid shift may appear volume overloaded (e.g., showing weight gain and edema) yet be clinically volume depleted (e.g., having symptoms of hypotension and tachycardia) because of a reduction in the effective circulating volume.

# Nursing Assessment of the Patient at Risk

## 4

Fluid and electrolyte homeostasis is essential for health and well-being. Unfortunately, fluid, electrolyte, and acid-base disturbances are potential complications of almost all disease states and medical therapies. Nurses in all areas of practice must be diligent in the assessment of individuals at risk for development of fluid, electrolyte, and acid-base disturbances. After an initial assessment and development of diagnoses, ongoing surveillance is critical to ensure adequate treatment or prevention of imbalances.

## Nursing History

Each of the following dimensions of the health history should be considered.

### Physiologic

Does the individual have any diseases or disorders that may cause a disturbance in fluid and electrolyte homeostasis (e.g., ulcerative colitis, diabetes mellitus)? Is the individual receiving any medications or therapy that may cause a disturbance in fluid, electrolyte, and acid-base status (e.g., diuretics, nasogastric [NG] suction)?

### Developmental

Is the individual at increased risk because of age or social situation (e.g., an older adult who lives alone)? NOTE: Fluid volume deficit is more common in infants and older adults (see Appendix C).

## Psychologic

Are there behavioral or emotional problems that may increase the risk of fluid, electrolyte, and acid-base disturbances (e.g., bulimia or noncompliance in the teenager with diabetes)?

## Spiritual

Does the individual have any beliefs, values, or practices that may affect the ability to comply with medical interventions (e.g., the Jehovah's Witness with gastrointestinal [GI] bleeding who refuses human blood products) or increase the risk for imbalance (e.g., religious fasting)?

## Sociocultural

Are there any social, cultural, financial, or educational factors that place the individual at increased risk or affect the ability to comply with medical therapy (e.g., the patient on a fixed income who, in an attempt to save money, fills only the digoxin and diuretic prescriptions but not the potassium supplement prescription)?

## Clinical Assessment

Two of the most important tools for the clinical assessment of fluid balance problems are simple nursing procedures that may be initiated without a physician's order: daily weights and intake and output (I&O). Hemodynamic monitoring is an invasive means of assessment of fluid balance disorders.

## Daily Weights

Acute weight changes are usually indicative of acute fluid changes. Each kilogram (kg) of weight lost or gained suggests 1 liter (L) of fluid lost or gained. Thus a 2-kg acute weight loss equals a 2-L fluid loss. Weight gains do not necessarily indicate an increase in effective circulating volume but rather an increase in total body volume that may be located in any of the fluid compartments. For accuracy and consistency, weight should be measured at the same time each day, preferably before breakfast. The scale should be balanced before each use, and the individual should be weighed wearing approximately the same clothing. The type of scale (i.e., standing, bed, chair) should be noted so that whenever possible the same scale can be used.

## Intake and Output

All I&O should be accurately measured whenever possible, with all unmeasured volumes estimated and noted. The I&O record should include the following:

1. **Intake**
   - *Oral fluids:* Ice chips must be included and recorded as fluids at approximately one half their volume. The nurse should include all foods that are liquid at room temperature.
   - *Parenteral fluids:* Parenteral fluid containers are often overfilled, and the excess should be discarded during setup or the exact amount given should be recorded.
   - *Tube feedings:* Often a 30-milliliter (mL) to 50-mL water flush is given at the end of intermittent tube feedings or periodically during continuous tube feedings. This flush needs to be included in the intake record.
   - *Catheter irrigants:* If the catheter is irrigated or lavaged and an equal amount is not withdrawn and discarded, the extra irrigant should be added to the intake record.
2. **Output**
   - *Urine output:* Ideally measured hourly.
   - *Liquid feces*
   - *Vomitus*
   - *NG drainage*
   - *Excessive sweating:* May be documented either via a rating system (e.g., 1+ for noticeable sweating to 4+ for profuse sweating) or by documenting the amount of linen saturated with sweat.
   - *Wound drainage:* May be documented by noting the type and number of dressings saturated, by weighing dressings, or by direct measurement of drainage contained in a gravity or vacuum drainage device (e.g., Hemovac, drainage bags).
   - *Draining fistulas:* If possible, drainage should be collected in a stoma bag or the amount of dressings or linen saturated should be documented.

■ *Rapid or labored respiratory rate:* Contributes to a patient's insensible fluid loss and should be documented.

## Hemodynamic Monitoring

Hemodynamic monitoring may be useful in evaluation of fluid volume abnormalities and certain acid-base disorders (Table 4-1).

1. **Central venous pressure (CVP):** Measurement of mean right atrial pressure and right ventricular end-diastolic pressure with a catheter that is inserted in or near the right atrium. A normal reading is 2 to 6 millimeters of mercury (mm Hg) or 5 to 12 centimeters of water (cm $H_2O$).
2. **Pulmonary artery pressure (PAP):** Measured with a catheter passed through the right heart and into the pulmonary artery (PA) with the tip positioned in the pulmonary capillary bed. Normal PAP is 20 to 30/8 to 15 mm Hg. PA diastolic pressures may be used to estimate left ventricular end-diastolic pressure and thus evaluate cardiac performance. In addition to measurement of cardiac and vascular pressures, specialized PA catheters allow measurement of cardiac output (CO) and mixed venous oxygen saturation, which may provide information about volume and acid-base status.

Table 4-1    Hemodynamic evaluation of fluid volume abnormalities

| Clinical Reading | Potential Cause |
|---|---|
| CVP <2 mm Hg or <5 cm $H_2O$ PAP <20/8 mm Hg | Decreased effective circulating volume resulting from true volume depletion (e.g., bleeding), shifting of fluid out of vascular space (e.g., burns), or vasodilation (e.g., after administration of certain antihypertensive medications) |
| CVP >6 mm Hg or >12 cm $H_2O$ | Fluid overload, poor right ventricular function, or constriction of pulmonary vascular bed |
| PAP >30/15 mm Hg | Increases in fluid volume or pulmonary vascular resistance |

# Vital Signs

The following examples are changes in vital signs that may signal fluid, electrolyte, or acid-base imbalance:

## Body Temperature

1. **Elevations in body temperature:** May lead to fluid and electrolyte losses as a result of increased insensible loss. Hypernatremic (elevated sodium) dehydration may cause an elevation in temperature.
2. **Decreases in body temperature:** May result from hypovolemia. With severe fluid volume deficit, the rectal temperature may drop to as low as 35° C (95° F).

## Respiratory Rate and Depth

1. **Increases in respiratory rate and depth:** Increase insensible fluid loss and may contribute to the development of volume depletion.
2. **Rapid, deep respirations:** May be compensating for metabolic acidosis.
3. **Shortness of breath, crackles (rales), or rhonchi:** May signal fluid buildup in the lungs caused by fluid volume excess.

## Heart Rate/Pulses

1. **Heart rate:** Increased heart rate may occur with fluid volume deficit as a compensatory mechanism for maintaining CO.
2. **Bounding pulse:** May signal fluid volume excess. The strength and volume of the pulse is dependent on the volume of blood ejected by the left ventricle and the strength of the left ventricular contraction. Both may increase in fluid volume excess.
3. **Weak, thready pulse:** May signal fluid volume deficit because of a reduction in intravascular volume.
4. **Irregular heart rate:** May occur with hypokalemia or hypomagnesemia from the development of dysrhythmias.

## Blood Pressure

Blood pressure (BP) is determined by multiplying CO by systemic vascular resistance. CO, in turn, is the product of heart rate multiplied by stroke volume (the amount of blood moved with each contraction of the left ventricle). Thus changes in stroke volume, heart rate, or vascular resistance may result in changes in BP.

1. **Decreased BP:** May signal fluid volume deficit from a reduction in stroke volume. Electrolyte imbalances that cause dysrhythmias may decrease BP if either heart rate or stroke volume is affected.

2. **Elevated BP:** May signal fluid volume excess because of an increase in stroke volume.

3. **Postural changes in BP or heart rate:** May be used to assess for fluid volume deficit. If on standing the systolic pressure decreases 20 mm Hg or more or the pulse increases 10 beats/minute or more from the value recorded while the patient was lying flat, orthostatic changes are present, suggesting inadequate intravascular fluid volume. Although orthostatic hypotension typically indicates the presence of fluid volume deficit, it may also be present in individuals with autonomic neuropathy from a variety of disorders, including diabetes. For accurate results, the individual should be lying flat for at least 2 minutes before measurement of supine BP and pulse and should remain standing for at least 1 minute before measurement of upright vital signs.

## Physical Assessment

The following are some examples of changes noted on physical assessment that may be indicative of fluid, electrolyte, or acid-base imbalance. (See the sections on individual fluid and electrolyte disorders in Chapters 6 through 11 and acid-base disorders in Chapters 12 through 17 for additional information.)

### Integumentary System

1. **Flushed, dry skin:** May signal fluid volume deficit.
2. **Changes in skin turgor:** May reflect changes in interstitial fluid (ISF) volume. Turgor may be assessed with pinching of the skin over the forearm, sternum, or dorsum of the hand. With adequate hydration, the pinched skin returns quickly to its original position when released. With fluid volume deficit, the pinched skin stays elevated for several seconds.

This is a less reliable indicator in older adults because of the skin's decreased elasticity. In these individuals, skin turgor is best assessed on the inner aspect of the thigh or over the sternum.

3. **Edema:** Indicates an expanded interstitial volume. Edema may be localized (usually the result of inflammation) or generalized (because of altered capillary hemodynamics and the retention of excess sodium and water) and usually is most evident in dependent areas. The presence of periorbital edema suggests significant fluid retention. Pitting should be assessed over a bony surface such as the tibia or sacrum and rated according to severity (e.g., 1+ for barely detectable edema to 4+ for deep, persistent pitting [see Figure 6-2]). (See Chapter 6 for additional information.)

4. **Increased furrowing of the tongue:** Suggestive of fluid volume deficit.

5. **Decreased moisture between the cheek and gum in the oral cavity:** Signals fluid volume deficit.

## Cardiovascular System

1. **Assessment of jugular venous distention:** Provides an estimate of CVP. With the head of the bed at a 30- to 45-degree angle, the distance between the level of the sternal angle (Louis' angle) and the point at which the internal and external jugular veins collapse is measured. Optimally this distance should be 3 centimeters (cm) or less (Figure 4-1). Values of greater than 3 cm suggest fluid volume excess or decreased cardiac function.

2. **Assessment of the veins of the hands:** May be used to assess fluid volume status. Normally, elevation of the hand collapses the veins in 3 to 5 seconds; lowering of the hand refills them in 3 to 5 seconds. With fluid volume deficit, the veins of the lowered hand need more than 3 to 5 seconds to fill. With fluid volume excess, the veins of the elevated hand need more than 3 to 5 seconds to empty.

3. **Assessment of heart sounds:** Development of an $S_3$ may indicate fluid volume excess.

4. **Dysrhythmias:** May occur with potassium, calcium, and magnesium abnormalities (see the individual sections in Chapters 8, 9, and 11 for a discussion of specific electrocardiogram changes).

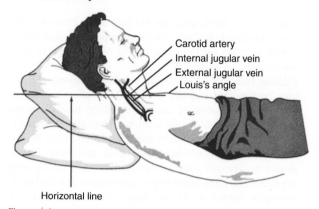

Carotid artery
Internal jugular vein
External jugular vein
Louis's angle

Horizontal line

Figure 4-1
**Inspection of external jugular venous pressure.**
(Modified from Thompson JM et al: *Mosby's clinical nursing,* ed 5, St Louis, 2002, Mosby.)

## Neurologic System

1. **Changes in level of consciousness (LOC):** Occur with changes in serum osmolality or changes in serum sodium. The severity of the symptoms depends on the rate and degree of change. Changes in LOC also may occur with acute acid-base imbalances.
2. **Restlessness and confusion:** May occur with fluid volume deficit or acid-base imbalance.
3. **Abnormal reflexes:** Occur with calcium and magnesium changes. Calcium and magnesium deficits enhance neuromuscular excitability (e.g., hyperactive reflexes), whereas calcium and magnesium excesses depress neuromuscular function (e.g., diminished reflexes).
4. **Positive Trousseau's sign and Chvostek's sign:** Can occur with hypocalcemia and hypomagnesemia.
   - *Positive Trousseau's sign:* Ischemia-induced carpal spasm, elicited with application of a BP cuff to the upper arm and inflation past systolic BP for 2 minutes.
   - *Positive Chvostek's sign:* Unilateral contraction of the facial and eyelid muscles, elicited with irritation of the facial nerve by percussing the face just in front of the ear.

5. **Neuromuscular changes resulting from altered membrane polarization of excitable tissue:** Caused by abnormalities in potassium or calcium levels. For example, neuromuscular symptoms of tingling, paresthesias, weakness, and flaccid paralysis may occur with hyperkalemia. Weakness, cramps, dysrhythmias, and paralysis may occur with hypokalemia. Neuromuscular irritability and paresthesias may also occur with metabolic and respiratory alkalosis.

## Gastrointestinal System

1. **Anorexia, nausea, and vomiting:** May occur with acute fluid volume deficit or fluid volume excess.
2. **Thirst:** Symptomatic of increased osmolality or fluid volume deficit.

# Laboratory Assessment of Fluid, Electrolyte, and Acid-Base Balance

5

Laboratory tests are vital in the early identification and continuous monitoring of fluid, electrolyte, and acid-base imbalances. Consideration of laboratory results should be included in the nursing assessment of patients at risk for fluid, electrolyte, and acid-base disturbances. The laboratory values that follow are applicable to adults.

## Tests to Evaluate Fluid Status
### Serum Osmolality

*Reference range: 280 to 300 milliosmoles/kg (mOsm/kg).*

Serum osmolality is the measurement of the number of osmotically active solutes in the serum. It may be measured directly, or it may be estimated with doubling the serum sodium because sodium and its accompanying anions are the primary determinants of serum osmolality. A more exact estimate of serum osmolality considers glucose and urea with the following formula:

Serum osmolality

$$= 2Na + \frac{\text{Serum glucose}}{18} + \frac{\text{Urea (blood urea nitrogen [BUN])}}{2.8}$$

Because glucose and urea are measured by weight (milligrams/deciliter [mg/dL]), those values must be converted to concentration (number of particles) by dividing the weight per liter (L) of solution by the molecular weight of each substance. Hence, glucose is divided by 18 and BUN is divided by 2.8.

1. **Factors that may increase serum osmolality:**
   - *Free water loss:* For example, increased insensible water loss (see Chapter 3 for a discussion of insensible water loss) or diabetes insipidus (see Chapter 20 for additional information).
   - *Sodium overload:* For example, excessive administration of sodium bicarbonate ($NaHCO_3$).
   - *Hyperglycemia:* See Chapter 20.
   - *Renal failure:* Caused by increased urea (see Chapter 22).

2. **Factors that may decrease serum osmolality:**
   - *Syndrome of inappropriate secretion of antidiuretic hormone (SIADH):* See Chapter 20.
   - *Diuretics*
   - *Adrenal insufficiency:* See the section on Addisonian Crisis in Chapter 20.
   - *Renal failure:* Caused by retention of excess water (see Chapter 22).
   - *Isotonic fluid loss:* Replaced with water or hypotonic fluids (e.g., vomiting of isotonic gastric contents with water replacement).

## Hematocrit

*Reference range: 40% to 54% (in males) and 37% to 47% (in females).*

Hematocrit measures the volume (percentage) of whole blood that is made up of red blood cells (RBCs). Because hematocrit measures the percentage of cells in relation to plasma, it is affected by changes in plasma volume. Thus the hematocrit increases with dehydration and decreases with overhydration. The hematocrit may be normal immediately after an acute hemorrhage (the concentration of RBCs to plasma has not changed), but over a period of hours, a shift of fluid from the interstitial fluid (ISF) to the plasma occurs and the hematocrit drops. In addition, the kidneys compensate for the loss of volume by retaining sodium and water.

## Urea Nitrogen

*Reference range: BUN is 6 to 20 mg/dL.*

Urea is produced as a byproduct of hepatic protein metabolism. Its primary means of removal from the body is excretion by the kidneys. Urea production occurs at a fairly steady rate so that increased BUN usually reflects a reduction in renal function. However, urea synthesis and excretion can be affected by additional factors such as hydration, protein intake, and tissue catabolism, thereby limiting the usefulness of BUN as an indicator of renal function.

1. **Factors that may increase BUN:**
   - *Decreased renal function:* If the increase in BUN is solely the result of reduced renal function, the serum creatinine level increases at approximately the same rate (BUN: creatinine ratio is 10:1 to 20:1).
   - *Excessive protein intake*
   - *Gastrointestinal (GI) bleeding:* From digestion of blood in the gut.
   - *Increased tissue catabolism (breakdown):* Occurs, for example, with fever, sepsis, or antianabolic steroid use.
   - *Volume depletion or other conditions that cause decreased renal perfusion (e.g., congestive heart failure [CHF]):* Because urea excretion varies with water excretion, conditions associated with increased renal resorption of water result in an increased BUN. In the presence of significant renal water conservation, the BUN:creatinine ratio increases (i.e., to >20:1).
2. **Factors that may decrease BUN:**
   - *Low-protein diet*
   - *Severe liver disease:* Caused by decreased hepatic synthesis.
   - *Volume expansion:* Occurs, for example, with overhydration with intravenous (IV) fluids or pregnancy.

## Urine Osmolality

*Physiologic range is approximately 50 to 1200 mOsm/kg; a typical 24-hour specimen is approximately 300 to 900 mOsm/kg.*

Urine osmolality is a measure of the solute concentration of the urine. Unlike plasma, the primary determinants of urinary osmolality are nitrogenous wastes (e.g., urea, creatinine, uric acid). The kidneys are capable of excreting concentrated, yet almost sodium-free, urine. Although the maximum urine osmolality in adults may be as high as 1200 mOsm/kg, the neonate is capable of concentrating urine to no greater than 500 mOsm/kg and the child to only 700 mOsm/kg.

It should be noted that urinary values for concentration and composition are normal or abnormal only in relation to what is occurring in the blood. A patient with severe diaphoresis, for example, is expected to have a relatively high urine osmolality (the kidneys should be compensating for the hypotonic fluid loss by retaining water). In contrast, a patient who has been overhydrated with IV 5% dextrose in water ($D_5W$) is expected to have a relatively low urine osmolality (the kidneys should be compensating for the excess water intake by excreting dilute urine). In this case, a relatively high urine osmolality is abnormal.

1. **Factors that may increase urine osmolality:**
   - *Fluid volume deficit*
   - *SIADH:* Urine osmolality is inappropriately high, given the serum osmolality (see Chapter 20).
2. **Factors that may decrease urine osmolality:**
   - *Fluid volume excess*
   - *Diabetes insipidus:* See Chapter 20 for additional information.

## Urine Specific Gravity

*Physiologic range is 1.001 to 1.040; random specimen with normal fluid intake is approximately 1.010 to 1.020.*

Specific gravity measures the weight of a solution in relation to water (water = 1.000). Urine specific gravity evaluates the kidneys' ability to conserve or excrete water. It is a less reliable indicator of concentration than urine osmolality because specific gravity is affected both by the weight and number of solutes. Depending on the testing method, the presence in the urine of a few large solutes such as glucose or protein may cause a deceptively high specific gravity. Advantages of the test are that it can be performed quickly, easily, and inexpensively at

Table 5-1 Relationship of osmolality to specific gravity

| Osmolality | Specific Gravity |
|---|---|
| 350 mOsm/kg | ≈1.010 |
| 700 mOsm/kg | ≈1.020 |
| 1050 mOsm/kg | ≈1.030 |
| 1400 mOsm/kg | ≈1.040 (physiologic maximum for urinary concentration) |

the bedside by nursing staff. (Table 5-1 shows the relationship of osmolality to specific gravity.)

Factors that increase and decrease specific gravity are the same as those that affect urine osmolality. Some substances that may give a false high specific gravity include glucose, protein, dextran, radiographic contrast material, and medications such as carbenicillin disodium. Children of less than age 2 years and older adults have a decreased ability to concentrate urine, so the upper limit of specific gravity is lower in these individuals.

## Urine Sodium

*Normal random specimen ranges from 50 to 130 milliequivalents (mEq)/L.*

Urine sodium levels vary with sodium intake (e.g., increased intake results in increased excretion) and volume status (e.g., sodium is conserved in the presence of a decreased effective circulating volume [ECV]). Levels may be measured from 24-hour specimens or random specimens.

It should be noted that diuretics and advanced renal failure might increase urine sodium levels.

**Clinical applications of urine sodium levels:**

- *Evaluation of volume status*
- *Differential diagnosis of hyponatremia (decreased serum sodium)*
- *Differential diagnosis of acute renal failure*

Urine sodium, osmolality, and specific gravity may be helpful in differentiating between oliguria caused by decreased ECV and oliguria from acute tubular necrosis (ATN). In volume depletion or decreased ECV, the kidneys are able to respond appropriately by conserving sodium and concentrating urine.

Table 5-2   Urinary values: hypovolemia versus acute tubular necrosis (ATN)

| Urinary Test | Hypovolemia | ATN |
|---|---|---|
| Urine osmolality (mOsm/kg of water) | > 350 | ≤350 |
| Urine specific gravity | 1.020 | Fixed at ≈1.010 |
| Urine sodium | < 20 | > 40 |
| $FE_{Na}$ | < 1% | > 1% |

Thus urine sodium is minimal, urine osmolality exceeds plasma osmolality, and urine specific gravity is greater than 1.015. In ATN (a type of acute renal failure [see Chapter 22]), the kidneys lose the ability to conserve sodium and concentrate urine appropriately. Urine osmolality remains fixed at less than 350 mOsm/kg, specific gravity is fixed at approximately 1.010, and urine sodium typically is greater than 20 to 40 mmol/L (Table 5-2).

Fractional excretion of sodium ($FE_{Na}$) is a calculation that may also help differentiate between decreased renal perfusion and ATN. It reports the percentage of filtered sodium that is excreted by the kidneys. Urine sodium, urine creatinine, serum sodium, and serum creatinine values are necessary to calculate $FE_{Na}$. As with urine sodium, $FE_{Na}$, is low (< 1%) in volume depletion and higher (> 2%) in ATN.

## Tests to Evaluate Electrolyte Balance

Refer to Chapters 7 through 11 for individual discussions of each of the electrolytes. (Table 5-3 provides the normal values.)

## Tests to Evaluate Acid-Base Balance
### Arterial Blood Gases

Arterial blood gases (ABGs) measure the pH, carbon dioxide ($CO_2$) tension, and oxygen ($O_2$) tension of arterial blood and the $O_2$ saturation of hemoglobin. A bicarbonate ($HCO_3^-$) level of arterial blood is also included in an ABG test and may be

Table 5-3    Serum electrolytes: normal ranges

| | |
|---|---|
| $Na^+$ | 135-145 mmol/L |
| $Cl^-$ | 95-108 mmol/L |
| Potassium | 3.5-5 mmol/L |
| Total $CO_2$ | 22-28 mmol/L |
| Calcium (total) | 8.5-10.5 mg/dl |
| | 4.3-5.3 mEq/L |
| Magnesium (total) | 1.8-3 mg/dl |
| | 1.5-2.5 mEq/L |
| Phosphorus | 2.5-4.5 mg/dl |
| | 1.7-2.6 mEq/L |

Table 5-4    Arterial blood gases: normal ranges

| | |
|---|---|
| pH | 7.35-7.45 |
| $Pa_{CO_2}$ | 35-45 mm Hg |
| $Pa_{O_2}$ | 80-95 mm Hg |
| $O_2$ saturation | 95%-99% |
| $HCO_3^-$ | 22-26 mmol/L |

*mm Hg*, Millimeters of mercury.

measured directly or calculated from pH and $CO_2$ tension of arterial blood ($Pa_{CO_2}$). ABGs evaluate acid-base balance and pulmonary function. (Table 5-4 lists normal ABG values. See Chapter 12 for additional information, including a step-by-step guide to ABG analysis.)

## Carbon Dioxide Content or Total Carbon Dioxide

*Reference range: 22 to 28 mmol/L.*

With a venous blood sample, this test measures $CO_2$ content in all its chemical forms: dissolved $CO_2$ ($P_{CO_2}$), $HCO_3^-$, and carbonic acid ($H_2CO_3$). $H_2CO_3$ exists only briefly; therefore its concentration is negligible. Because dissolved $CO_2$ accounts for only 1.2 mmol/L, the $CO_2$ content primarily reflects the $HCO_3^-$ level. The $CO_2$ increases in metabolic alkalosis and decreases in metabolic acidosis.

## Anion Gap

*Reference range: 10 to 14 mmol/L.*

Anion gap is a calculated value that reflects the normally unmeasured anions (e.g., phosphates, sulfates, proteins) in the plasma. Anion gap equals sodium ($Na^+$) − (chloride [$Cl^-$] + $HCO_3^-$). Measurement of the anion gap (Figure 5-1) may be helpful in the differential diagnosis of metabolic acidosis or in identification of hidden metabolic acidosis in certain mixed acid-base disorders (see Chapters 15 through 17).

To understand anion gap, think of the extracellular fluid (ECF) as two equal-sized columns—one containing cations (positively charged ions) and the other containing anions (negatively charged ions). Because electroneutrality is maintained at all times within the body, the number of cations and anions (or the size of the two columns as shown in Figure 5-1) must always be equal. Sodium is the body's primary cation; thus the overall size of column 1 may be determined with measurement of serum sodium. The two primary anions of the ECF are $Cl^-$ and $HCO_3^-$. Their sum ($Cl^-$ mmol/L + $HCO_3^-$ mmol/L) does not completely fill column 2. The remaining portion of column 2 represents the normally unmeasured anions of the ECF or anion gap. The anion gap is calculated from a serum electrolyte panel with the following formula:

$$\text{Anion gap (mystery box)} = Na^+ - (Cl^- + HCO_3^-)$$

The size of anion gap is significant because the main causes of metabolic acidosis fall into two categories: 1, those that cause an increase in unmeasured anions and thus increase the mystery box/anion gap; and 2, those that result from a loss of $HCO_3^-$ or an ingestion or administration of acidifying salts and do not alter the mystery box/anion gap. (See Boxes 5-1 and 5-2 and Chapters 15 and 17 for additional information.)

## Urine pH

*Reference range for a random specimen: 4.6 to 8.*

The kidneys play a critical role in the regulation of acid-base balance by excreting a portion of the hydrogen ions ($H^+$) produced each day. Despite a buffering system within the renal

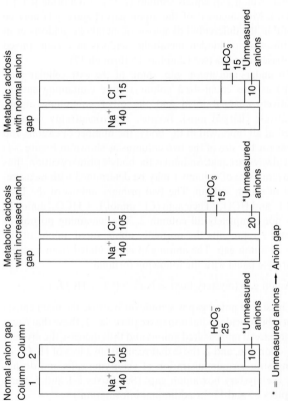

Figure 5-1
Anion gap and metabolic acidosis.

## Box 5-1 Causes of Metabolic Acidosis with a Normal Anion Gap

Loss of Bicarbonate

- Diarrhea
- Lower GI fistulas
- Ureterosigmoidostomy
- Renal tubular acidosis
- Early renal insufficiency
- Diuretics: acetazolamide (Diamox), triamterene (Dyrenium), spironolactone (Aldactone)

Addition of Acidifying Salts

- Ammonium chloride
- Hyperalimentation fluids without adequate $HCO_3^-$ or $HCO_3^-$-producing solutes (e.g., lactate, acetate)
- Lysine hydrochloride
- Arginine hydrochloride

## Box 5-2 Causes of Metabolic Acidosis with an Increased Anion Gap

Retention of Acids

- Renal failure

Ingestion

- Salicylates
- Methanol
- Paraldehyde

Abnormal Production of Acids

- Ketoacidosis
- Lactic acidosis

tubule, which allows maximal excretion of $H^+$ with minimal decrease in urinary pH, the pH of the urine usually is markedly acidic (averaging approximately 6). Measurement of urine pH may be useful in determination of whether the kidneys are responding appropriately to metabolic acid-base imbalances. Urine pH should decrease in metabolic acidosis and increase in metabolic alkalosis. An inappropriately high urine pH in the presence of metabolic acidosis, for example, suggests renal tubular acidosis (a group of disorders that inhibit renal excretion of $H^+$). An inappropriately low pH in the presence of metabolic alkalosis may signal volume depletion (i.e., $NaHCO_3$ is retained as the kidneys attempt to correct the volume deficit by conserving all filtered sodium). Urinary tract infections with pathogens that produce urease cause alkaline urine because of excess ammonia production. Urine pH should be measured within 1 to 2 hours of collection. Urine becomes increasingly alkaline as it sits.

## Lactate

*Reference range venous specimen: 0.7 to 2.1 mEq/L.*

Lactic acid is a byproduct of the anaerobic metabolism of glucose. Normally, the small quantity of lactic acid that is produced daily is immediately buffered by $HCO_3^-$ and lactate is generated. This lactate is then converted to $CO_2$ and water or glucose by the liver, and $HCO_3^-$ is regenerated. Any time there is an excess production of lactic acid (e.g., when there is a decreased $O_2$ delivery to the tissue) or decreased utilization of lactate dangerous lactic acidosis may develop.

1. **Factors that may lead to the development of lactic acidosis:**
   - *Increased production of lactic acid:*
     Strenuous exercise
     Shock/sepsis
     Cardiac arrest
     Carbon monoxide poisoning
     Hypoxemia
   - *Decreased utilization of lactate:*
     Liver disease
     Severe acidosis

# Related Tests
## Creatinine

*Reference range: 0.6 to 1.5 mg/dL.*

Creatinine is a metabolic waste product produced by the breakdown of muscle creatine. The serum creatinine level reflects the balance between production and excretion by the kidneys. Because it is produced at a steady rate dependent on muscle mass and is not affected by diet, hydration, or tissue catabolism, the creatinine level is a more accurate indicator of renal function than BUN. The serum creatinine level increases as renal function decreases. Small changes in creatinine may reflect a significant alteration in renal function.

## Serum Albumin

*Reference range: 3.5 to 5.5 grams (g)/dL.*

Albumin is a small plasma protein produced by the liver that acts osmotically to help hold the intravascular volume in the vascular space. Decreased serum albumin (hypoalbuminemia) may lead to the development of edema as a result of the movement of water out of the vascular space and into the interstitial space. The edema seen in protein malnutrition occurs as a result of decreased albumin production.

**Factors that may decrease serum albumin:**
- *Decreased protein intake (e.g., protein malnutrition)*
- *Decreased hepatic synthesis (e.g., cirrhosis)*
- *Abnormal urinary loss (e.g., nephrotic syndrome)*

# DISORDERS OF FLUID, ELECTROLYTE, AND ACID-BASE BALANCE

## II

# Disorders of Fluid Balance

6

## Hypovolemia

Depletion of extracellular fluid (ECF) volume is termed *hypovolemia*. Hypovolemia occurs because of abnormal skin, gastrointestinal (GI), or renal losses; bleeding; decreased intake; or movement of fluid into a nonequilibrating third space (Table 6-1). Depending on the type of fluid lost, hypovolemia may be accompanied by acid-base, osmolar, or electrolyte imbalances. Severe ECF volume depletion can lead to hypovolemic shock. Compensatory mechanisms in hypovolemia include increased sympathetic nervous system stimulation (increased heart rate [HR], inotropy [cardiac contraction], and vascular resistance), thirst, release of antidiuretic hormone (ADH), and release of aldosterone. Prolonged hypovolemia may lead to the development of acute renal failure (see Chapter 22).

## Assessment

1. **Clinical manifestations:** Dizziness, weakness, fatigue, syncope, anorexia, nausea, vomiting, thirst, confusion, constipation, and oliguria.
2. **Physical assessment:** Decreased blood pressure (BP), especially when standing (orthostatic hypotension); increased HR; dry, furrowed tongue; sunken eyeballs; flattened neck veins; increased temperature; and acute weight loss (Table 6-2), except with third spacing.
   - *Infants and children:* Loss of tearing, depressed anterior fontanelle, and poor skin turgor.

   The patient in shock appears pale and diaphoretic with a rapid, thready pulse; the patient has supine hypotension, oliguria, and confusion. (Box 6-1 lists assessment changes associated with hypovolemia.)

55

Table 6-1    Common disorders associated with third-space fluid shift*

| Disorder | Pathophysiologic Process |
|---|---|
| Peritonitis | Trapping of fluid and electrolytes in peritoneal cavity, owing to damage to or inflammation of peritoneum. As many as 6 L of fluid can accumulate, depending on degree of acuity. |
| Bowel obstruction | Loss of lower GI fluid caused by sequestering of GI fluid in distended bowel. Several liters may accumulate in intestinal lumen, leading to dramatic increase in lumen pressure with eventual damage to intestinal mucosa. |
| Burns | Temporary sequestering of fluid in interstitial space from increased capillary permeability and decreased vascular colloid osmotic pressure. |
| Ascites | Accumulation of several liters of fluid in peritoneal cavity, occurring in severe hepatic cirrhosis. Ascites occurs in cirrhosis as result of hepatic venous obstruction and retention of sodium and water. Symptomatic hypovolemia is most likely to occur after paracentesis because of rapid reaccumulation of ascitic fluid. |
| Fractured hip | Loss of intravascular volume caused by extensive bleeding into joint. |
| Carcinoma | Trapping of fluid in interstitial space caused by lymphatic or venous obstruction. |
| Major surgery involving extensive tissue trauma | Abnormal sequestration of fluid at surgical site because of extensive tissue involvement (e.g., with major abdominal surgery). It can also occur with loss of ECF into wall and lumen of bowel during bowel surgery. |

*There is no third space per se. Rather, it is a concept describing fluid that is temporarily unavailable either to ICF or ECF. Because third-space fluids are unavailable to the body for its use, the patient exhibits clinical indicators associated with fluid volume deficit (except for weight loss).

Table 6-2   Weight loss as an indicator of extracellular fluid deficit in adults and children

| Acute Weight Loss | Severity of Deficit |
| --- | --- |
| 2%-5% | Mild |
| 5%-10% | Moderate |
| 10%-15% | Severe |
| 15%-20% | Fatal |

| Box 6-1 | Assessment Changes with Hypovolemia | |
| --- | --- | --- |
| Mild Hypovolemia | Moderate Hypovolemia | Severe Hypovolemia |
| Anorexia | Orthostatic | Supine hypotension |
| Fatigue | hypotension | Rapid, thready pulse |
| Weakness | Tachycardia | Cool, clammy skin |
| | Decreased CVP | Oliguria |
| | Decreased | Confusion, stupor, |
| | urine output | coma |
| | Reduced tears | Absent tears |
| | Soft fontanelle | Sunken fontanelle |

3. **Hemodynamic measurements:** Decreased central venous pressure (CVP), decreased pulmonary artery pressure (PAP), decreased cardiac output (CO), decreased mean arterial pressure (MAP), and increased systemic vascular resistance (SVR).
4. History and risk factors:
   - *Abnormal GI losses:*
     Vomiting
     Nasogastric (NG) suctioning
     Diarrhea and intestinal drainage
   - *Abnormal skin losses:*
     Excessive diaphoresis from fever or exercise, burns, or cystic fibrosis
   - *Abnormal renal losses:*
     Diuretic therapy
     Diabetes insipidus

Renal disease (polyuric forms)
Adrenal insufficiency
Osmotic diuresis (e.g., uncontrolled diabetes mellitus, postdye study). (See p. 12 for a discussion of osmotic diuresis.)

- *Third spacing or plasma-to-interstitial fluid (ISF) shift:*
Peritonitis
Intestinal obstruction
Burns
Ascites (see Table 6-1)
- *Hemorrhage*
- *Altered intake:*
Coma
Fluid deprivation

## Diagnostic Tests

1. **Blood urea nitrogen (BUN):** Is increased from increased renal resorption of urea. Urea resorption increases because of a compensatory increase in the resorption of sodium and water. It may also be increased as a result of increased production (from increased tissue catabolism or GI bleeding) or decreased excretion (from decreased renal perfusion).
2. **BUN:creatinine ratio:** Is greater than 20:1. An equal rise in both BUN and creatinine (10:1 to 20:1) reflects a change in renal function, and a proportionately greater rise in BUN suggests volume depletion or increased production.
3. **Hematocrit:** Elevated with dehydration because of hemoconcentration; decreased in the presence of bleeding. The hematocrit remains normal immediately after acute hemorrhage, but over a period of hours there is a shift of fluid from the ISF to the plasma and the hematocrit drops (Figure 6-1).
4. **Serum electrolytes:** Variable, depending on type of fluid lost. Hypokalemia often occurs with abnormal GI or renal losses. Hyperkalemia occurs with adrenal insufficiency. Hypernatremia may be seen with increased insensible or sweat losses and diabetes insipidus. Hyponatremia occurs in most types of hypovolemia because of increased thirst and ADH release, which leads to increased water intake and retention, thus diluting the serum sodium. (See the discussions of individual electrolyte disorders in Chapters 7 through 11.)

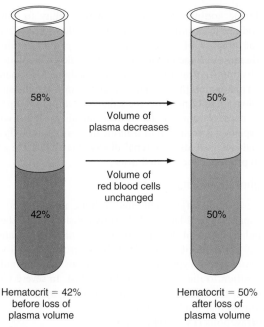

Figure 6-1
Example of acute effect of plasma volume loss on hematocrit.

5. **Serum osmolality:** Variable, depending on the type of fluid lost and the body's ability to compensate with thirst and increased production of ADH.
6. **Serum total carbon dioxide ($CO_2$) content (also termed $CO_2$ content):** Decreased with metabolic acidosis and increased with metabolic alkalosis (see the subsequent section on ABG values).
7. **Arterial blood gas (ABG) values:** Metabolic acidosis (pH < 7.35 and $HCO_3^-$ < 22 milliequivalents/liter [mmol/L]) may occur with lower GI losses, shock, or diabetic ketoacidosis. Metabolic alkalosis (pH > 7.45 and $HCO_3^-$ > 26 mmol/L) may occur with upper GI losses or diuretic therapy.
8. **Urine specific gravity:** Increased because of the kidneys' attempt to save water; may be fixed at approximately 1.010 in the presence of renal disease; is decreased with diabetes insipidus.

9. **Urine sodium**: Shows the kidneys' ability to conserve sodium in response to an increased aldosterone level. In the absence of renal disease, osmotic diuresis, diuretic therapy, or hypoaldosteronism, it should be less than 10 to 20 mmol/L. Fractional excretion of sodium is less than 1%.

10. **Urine osmolality:** Usually greater than 450 milliosmoles/kilogram (mOsm/kg) as the kidneys attempt to compensate by conserving water. The urine osmolality is less if volume depletion is the result of osmotic diuresis, diuretic therapy, diabetes insipidus, or renal disease that limits the ability to produce concentrated urine.

## Collaborative Management

For restoration of normal fluid volume and correction of accompanying acid-base and electrolyte disturbances, the type of fluid replacement depends on the type of fluid lost and the severity of the deficit; serum electrolytes; serum osmolality; and acid-base status. Typically, the replacement fluid is similar in composition to the type of fluid that is lost. In severe volume depletion, the initial goal of replacement is rapid restoration of intravascular fluid (IVF) volume.

1. **Intravenous (IV) fluid therapy**
   *Crystalloid solutions*
   - *Isotonic (normal) saline:* Expands ECF only; does not enter ICF; usually used as an intravascular volume expander or to replace abnormal losses.
   - *Saline/electrolyte solutions:* Provide additional electrolytes (e.g., potassium, calcium) and a buffer (e.g., lactate, acetate). Usually hypotonic solutions are used as maintenance fluids, whereas isotonic solutions are used as replacement fluids, because most abnormal fluid losses are isotonic.
   - *Dextrose and water:* Provides free water only and is distributed evenly throughout both intracellular fluid (ICF) and ECF; used to treat total body water deficits only.

   *Colloid solutions*
   - *Blood and blood components:* Expand only the intravascular portion of ECF.
   - *Plasma substitutes:* Dextran or hetastarch; expand the intravascular portion of ECF.

   (See Tables 6-3 and 6-4 and the section on Fluid Therapy for additional information.)

Table 6-3  Composition and use of commonly prescribed crystalloid solutions

| Solution | Glucose (g/L) | Electrolyte-Composition mmol/L | | | | Tonicity/mOsm/L | Indications and Considerations |
|---|---|---|---|---|---|---|---|
| | | $Na^+$ | $K^+$ | $Ca^{2+}$ | $Cl^-$ | $HCO_3^-$ | | |

| Solution | Glucose (g/L) | $Na^+$ | $K^+$ | $Ca^{2+}$ | $Cl^-$ | $HCO_3^-$ | Tonicity/mOsm/L | Indications and Considerations |
|---|---|---|---|---|---|---|---|---|
| **Dextrose in Water** | | | | | | | | |
| 1. 5% | 50 | — | — | — | — | — | Isotonic/252 | ■ Provides free water necessary for renal excretion of solutes<br>■ Used to replace water losses and treat hypernatremia<br>■ Used to administer variety of medications<br>■ Provides 170 kcal/L<br>■ Does not provide any electrolytes |
| 2. 10% | 100 | — | — | — | — | — | Hypertonic/505 | ■ Provides free water only, with no electrolytes<br>■ Provides 340 kcal/L |

*Continued*

Table 6-3   Composition and use of commonly prescribed crystalloid solutions—cont'd

| Solution | Glucose (g/L) | Electrolyte-Composition mmol/L. | | | | | Tonicity/mOsm/L. | Indications and Considerations |
| | | $Na^+$ | $K^+$ | $Ca^{2+}$ | $Cl^-$ | $HCO_3^-$ | | |
| --- | --- | --- | --- | --- | --- | --- | --- | --- |
| Saline | | | | | | | | |
| 3. 0.45% | — | 77 | — | — | 77 | — | Hypotonic/154 | ■ Provides free water in addition to $Na^+$ and $Cl^-$ ■ Used to replace hypotonic fluid losses ■ Used as maintenance solution, but does not replace daily losses of other electrolytes ■ Provides no calories ■ Can cause intravascular overload if infused too rapidly |
| 4. 0.9% | — | 154 | — | — | 154 | — | Isotonic/308 | ■ Used to expand intravascular volume and replace ECF losses; used as perioperative fluid |

|  |  |  |  |  | Tonicity/mOsm |  |
|---|---|---|---|---|---|---|
|  |  |  |  |  |  | - Only solution that may be administered with blood products |
|  |  |  |  |  |  | - Contains $Na^+$ and $Cl^-$ in excess of plasma levels |
|  |  |  |  |  |  | - Does not provide free water, calories, or other electrolytes |
|  |  |  |  |  |  | - May cause intravascular overload or hyperchloremic acidosis |
| 5. 3.0% | — | 513 | 513 | — | Hypertonic/1026 | - Used to treat symptomatic hyponatremia |
|  |  |  |  |  |  | - Must be administered slowly and with extreme caution because it may cause dangerous intravascular volume overload and pulmonary edema |
| Dextrose in Saline |  |  |  |  |  |  |
| 6. 5% in 0.225% | 50 | 38.5 | 38.5 | — | Isotonic/330 | - Provides $Na^+$, $Cl^-$, and free water |

*Continued*

Table 6-3   Composition and use of commonly prescribed crystalloid solutions—cont'd

| Solution | Glucose (g/L) | Electrolyte-Composition mmol/L | | | | | Tonicity/mOsm/L | Indications and Considerations |
|---|---|---|---|---|---|---|---|---|
| | | $Na^+$ | $K^+$ | $Ca^{2+}$ | $Cl^-$ | $HCO_3^-$ | | |
| 7. 5% in 0.45% | 50 | 77 | — | — | 77 | — | Hypertonic/406 | ■ Used to replace hypotonic losses and treat hypernatremia<br>■ Provides 170 kcal/L<br>■ Same as 0.45% NaCl, except that it provides 170 kcal/L |
| 8. 5% in 0.9% | 50 | 154 | — | — | 154 | — | Hypertonic/560 | ■ Same as 0.9% NaCl, except that it provides 170 kcal/L |
| **Multiple Electrolyte Solutions** | | | | | | | | |
| 9. Ringer's | — | 147 | 4 | 5 | 156 | — | Isotonic/309 | ■ Similar in composition to plasma, except that it has excess $Cl^-$, no $Mg^{2+}$, and no $HCO_3^-$<br>■ Does not provide free water or calories |

| 10. Lactated Ringer's (Hartmann's) solution | — | 130 | 4 | 3 | 109 | 28[*] | Isotonic/273 | ■ Used to expand intravascular volume and replace ECF losses<br>■ Similar in composition to normal plasma, except that it does not contain $Mg^{2+}$<br>■ Used to treat losses from burns and lower GI tract; used as perioperative fluid<br>■ May be used to treat mild metabolic acidosis; should not be used to treat lactic acidosis<br>■ Does not provide free water or calories |

Modified from Rose DB: *Clinical pathology of acid-base and electrolyte disorders*, ed 3, New York, 1989, McGraw-Hill Book.

[*]In the form of lactate.

Table 6-4   Composition and use of commonly prescribed colloid solutions

| Solution | Composition | Volume | Indications and Considerations |
|---|---|---|---|
| **Blood and Blood Components** | | | |
| Whole blood | RBCs, WBCs, platelets, plasma, and some clotting factors | Approximately 500 mL/unit | ■ Used to treat acute massive blood loss, although rarely necessary because most hemorrhagic episodes may be treated with packed RBCs and crystalloids<br>■ In stable patient, should increase hematocrit 3% or hemoglobin 1 g/dL/unit<br>■ Requires ABO and Rh compatibility<br>■ Administered with 0.9% NaCl only |
| Packed RBCs | RBCs and some plasma ($\approx$20%), platelets, and WBCs | 250-350 mL/unit | ■ Indicated in patients who need increased oxygen-carrying capacity but not necessarily volume expansion |

| | | | Less plasma proteins and clotting factors than whole blood<br>■ Requires ABO and Rh compatibility<br>■ Specially prepared leukocyte-depleted units may be used to decrease risk of febrile, nonhemolytic transfusion reactions<br>■ After 5 days, may have a potassium level of 20-30 mmol/L. Massive blood transfusions may cause hyperkalemia. |
|---|---|---|---|
| Fresh frozen plasma | Plasma, plasma proteins, and clotting factors | 200 mL | ■ Used to restore clotting factors in situations of known deficiency<br>■ Although helpful in restoring volume, should not be used solely for volume expansion |

*Continued*

Table 6-4 Composition and use of commonly prescribed colloid solutions—cont'd

| Solution | Composition | Volume | Indications and Considerations |
|---|---|---|---|
| Plasma protein fraction | 5% solution of human plasma proteins (85% albumin, 15% globulins) | 250-500 mL units 290 mOsm/L | ■ Should be used promptly after thawing to prevent deterioration of clotting factors<br>■ Requires ABO compatibility<br>■ Used to expand plasma volume<br>■ Has greater risk of hypersensitivity reactions than with pure albumin solutions |
| Albumin | Human albumin in buffered saline solution; available in 5% or 25% concentrations | 5% = 250 and 300 mL units 300 mOsm/L<br>25% = 50 and 100 mL units 1500 mOsm/L | ■ Does not require typing<br>■ Has virtually no risk of hepatitis or HIV infection<br>■ Used to expand plasma volume and increase plasma oncotic pressure<br>■ 25% albumin expands vascular volume 3 to 4 mL for each mL administered |

| | | |
|---|---|---|
| | | ■ Does not require typing |
| | | ■ Virtually no risk of hepatitis or HIV infection |
| | | ■ 25% should be used with caution in persons with cardiac or renal failure because of risk of IVF overload |
| **Plasma Substitutes** | | |
| Dextran 70 | 6% solution of polysaccharide (average molecular weight of 70,000) combined with saline or dextrose and water | 500 mL/unit |
| | | ■ Used for rapid volume expansion |
| | | ■ Less expensive than blood products |
| | | ■ May cause bleeding tendencies, interference with crossmatching, and release of histamine |

*Continued*

Table 6-4  Composition and use of commonly prescribed colloid solutions—cont'd

| Solution | Composition | Volume | Indications and Considerations |
|---|---|---|---|
| Hetastarch | 6% solution of hydroxyethyl starch in saline | 500 mL/unit 310 mOsm/L | ■ Used for rapid volume expansion<br>■ Less expensive than blood products<br>■ May cause bleeding tendencies and circulatory overload<br>■ Should be used with caution in persons with renal failure because of decreased urinary excretion of hetastarch |

*ABO*, Blood group system consisting of A, AB, B, and O; *HIV*, human immunodeficiency virus; *Rh*, rhesus factor; *WBCs*, white blood cells.

Fluids should be administered rapidly enough and in sufficient quantity to maintain adequate tissue perfusion without overloading the cardiovascular system. The patient's underlying cardiac and renal functions determine how well fluid replacement is tolerated. Thus the rate of fluid administration should be based on both severity of the loss and the individual's hemodynamic response to volume replacement. During a fluid challenge, volumes of fluid are administered at specific rates and intervals, and the patient's hemodynamic response is monitored and documented. Hemodynamic parameters may be prescribed by the physician or, depending on agency policy, determined with a fluid challenge protocol. A typical fluid challenge includes the following steps:

- Baseline vital signs (VS), hemodynamic measurements (e.g., CVP, PAP, CO), and clinical data (e.g., breath sounds, skin color and temperature, sensorium) are obtained.
- Initial volume of fluid is administered as prescribed or per protocol (e.g., 100 to 200 milliliters [mL] 0.9% sodium chloride [NaCl] over 10 minutes).
- The patient is reassessed after 10 minutes.
- If the patient continues to show signs of hypovolemia (i.e., CVP and PAP remain low), additional fluid may be administered per the physician or agency protocol.
- If the CVP or PAP increases too rapidly (e.g., >2 millimeters of mercury [mm Hg] for the CVP or >3 mm Hg for the PAP), fluid administration is discontinued and the patient is reassessed after 10 minutes. If after 10 minutes the CVP or PAP has dropped and the patient shows no signs of fluid overload, fluid administration is resumed.
- Fluid administration is continued until the desired hemodynamic parameters are achieved or a specific volume has been infused (e.g., 500 to 1000 mL). The fluid challenge should be discontinued if the patient shows signs of fluid volume excess (e.g., crackles [rales], increased HR, increased respiratory rate [RR]) or a rapid increase in CVP or PAP is seen.

NOTE: Continued nursing surveillance is essential during and after the fluid challenge.

2. **Restoration of tissue perfusion in hypovolemic shock:** The potential for the development of shock is dependent

on both the volume lost (usually > 25% of the intravascular volume) and the rapidity of the loss. In turn, successful treatment depends on rapid volume replacement. Initially, shock is treated with an isotonic electrolyte solution. A balanced electrolyte solution (e.g., Ringer's lactate) may be preferred because 0.9% NaCl contains excessive amounts of sodium and chloride (see Table 6-3). Hyperchloremic acidosis often develops after administration of large volumes of 0.9% NaCl. The clinical significance of iatrogenic hyperchloremic acidosis, however, remains questionable. Isotonic solutions distribute freely throughout the entire extracellular space, so that both the intravascular and interstitial spaces are expanded. Colloids such as human albumin, dextran, or hetastarch (see Table 6-4) also may be used to maximize intravascular volume expansion with less expansion of the ISF space. Their use, however, remains controversial because of cost, effectiveness, and potential side effects. Solutions that more closely approximate the fluid that was lost are used once tissue perfusion has been restored. In hemorrhagic shock, packed red blood cells (RBCs) are given as the hematocrit drops. Fresh frozen plasma is used to replace clotting factors when clotting disorders are present or massive transfusions are necessary. Autotransfusion has become an increasingly common therapy in hemorrhagic shock. Autologous blood drained from a sterile body cavity is retransfused within 4 hours of collection via an auto-transfusion device. Vasopressors may be used to augment volume restoration if endotoxic, anaphylactic, or neurogenic shock is also present.

3. **Oral rehydration:** Oral rehydration solutions (ORS) have been developed to treat mild to moderate fluid deficit associated with diarrhea or vomiting, common sources of abnormal fluid loss in infancy and early childhood. These solutions contain varying amounts of glucose, sodium, and potassium and some form of buffer. The glucose concentration of ORS is significant because of the relationship of glucose and sodium resorption in the gut. Maximal sodium and water absorption is believed to occur with glucose concentrations of 10 to 25 grams (g)/L. Commonly available fluids, such as "flat" cola drinks or ginger ale

and sports drinks, often are prescribed to replace fluids lost in mild episodes of diarrhea. However, these are poor choices for fluid replacement in prolonged or severe diarrhea because of the high glucose and low electrolyte concentrations (Table 6-5). (Table 6-6 provides examples of ORS.) Commercial ORS are now readily available in pharmacies and markets for home use. However, caregivers must be given explicit instructions concerning the use of ORS. Too-rapid administration may cause gastric distention with reflex vomiting. Initially, vomiting should be treated with 5 to 10 mL of ORS every 5 to 10 minutes. The volume may be increased gradually, as tolerated. In children, the fluid lost from each diarrheal stool should be replaced with ORS at a rate of 10 mL per kilogram of body weight.

4. **Hypodermoclysis:** This is the subcutaneous infusion of fluids typically used to treat dehydration in older adults, especially in long-term care facilities. Electrolyte-free and hypertonic fluids are not well tolerated.

5. **Treatment of the underlying cause:** In the case of hemorrhage, early operative treatment may improve survival.

## Nursing Diagnoses and Interventions

**Deficient fluid volume** related to abnormal loss of body fluids or reduced intake.

**Desired outcomes:** The patient attains adequate intake of fluid and electrolytes as evidenced by a urine output of greater than 0.5 mL/kg/hour, stable weight, specific gravity of 1.010 to 1.020, no clinical evidence of hypovolemia (e.g., furrowed tongue), BP within the patient's normal range, CVP of 2 to 6 mm Hg, and HR of 60 to 100 beats per minute (bpm). Serum sodium is 135 to 145 mmol/L, and hematocrit and BUN are within the patient's normal range. For patients in critical care, the following measurements are attained: PAP 20 to 30/8 to 15 mm Hg and CO 4 to 7 L/minute.

1. Monitor intake and output (I&O) hourly. Initially, intake should exceed output during therapy. Alert the physician to a urine output of less than 0.5 mL/kg/hour for 2 consecutive hours. Measure urine specific gravity every 4 to 8 hours; it should decrease with therapy.

Table 6-5  Composition of common clear liquids

| | Na$^+$ (mmol/L) | K$^+$ (mmol/L) | Cl$^-$ (mmol/L) | Base (mmol/L) | Osmolality (mOsm/L) | Carbohydrate (g/L) |
|---|---|---|---|---|---|---|
| Cola | 2 | 0 | 2 | 13 | 750 | 120 |
| Apple juice | 3 | 28 | 30 | 0 | 730 | 120 |
| Chicken broth | 250 | 8 | 250 | 0 | 450 | 0 |
| Gatorade | 23 | 3 | 17 | 3 | 330 | 46 |
| Tea | 0 | 5 | 0 | 0 | 5 | 0 |
| Ginger ale | 9 | 0.1 | 0 | 3.6 | 565 | 9 |
| Orange juice | 0.2 | 49 | 0 | 50 | 654 | 10.4 |

From Pflederer TA: Emergency fluid management of hypovolemia, *Postgrad Med* 100(3):243-254, 1996.

Table 6-6  Oral rehydration solutions

| | K cal/mL N (kcal/oz) | Carbohydrate (g/L) | Na (mEq/L) | K (mEq/L) | Osmolality (mOsm/kg H$_2$O) |
|---|---|---|---|---|---|
| Ceralyte-70 (Cera) | 0.16 (4.9) | Rice digest 40 | 70 | 20 | 232 |
| Ceralyte-50 (Cera) | 0.16 (4.9) | Rice digest, Glucose 40 | 50 | 20 | 200 |
| Enfalyte (Mead Johnson) | 0.12 (3.7) | Rice syrup solids 30 | 50 | 25 | 200 |
| Oral Rehydration Salts (WHO) (Jianas) | 0.06 (2) | Dextrose 20 | 90 | 20 | 330 |
| Pedialyte Unflavored (Ross) | 0.1 (3) | Dextrose 25 | 45 | 20 | 250 |
| Rehydralyte (Ross) | 0.1 (3) | Dextrose 25 | 75 | 20 | 305 |

From Gunn VL, Nechyba C: *The Harriet Lane handbook: a manual for pediatric house officers*, ed 16, St Louis, 2002, Mosby.

2. Monitor VS and hemodynamic pressures for signs of continued hypovolemia. Be alert to decreased BP and CVP and increased HR and SVR. For critical patients, also be alert to decreased PAP, CO, and MAP and increased SVR.

3. Weigh the patient daily. Daily weights are the single most important indicator of fluid status because acute weight changes usually indicate fluid changes. For example, in the individual who is being fed, a decrease in weight of 1 kg is equal to the loss of 1 L of fluid. Keep in mind, however, that the adult who is not eating or receiving any enteral or parenteral nutrition loses 0.25 kg of weight daily from actual loss of body tissue. Weigh the patient at the same time of day (preferably before breakfast) on a balanced scale, with the patient wearing approximately the same clothing. Document the type of scale used (i.e., standing, bed, chair).

4. Administer oral and IV fluids as prescribed. Document response to fluid therapy. Monitor for signs and symptoms of fluid overload or too-rapid fluid administration: crackles, shortness of breath (SOB), tachypnea, tachycardia, increased CVP, increased PAP, neck vein distention, and edema. If the patient has any of the previously mentioned signs and symptoms, consult with the physician.

5. Monitor the patient for hidden fluid losses. For example, measure and document abdominal girth or limb size if indicated.

6. Consult the physician for decreases in hematocrit that may signal bleeding. Remember that hematocrit decreases in a dehydrated patient as rehydration occurs. Decreases in hematocrit associated with rehydration may be accompanied by decreases in serum sodium and BUN.

7. Place the shock patient in a supine position with the legs elevated 45 degrees to increase venous return. This position returns approximately 500 mL of blood pooled in the veins of the legs to the central circulation. Avoid the Trendelenburg position because this causes abdominal viscera to press on the diaphragm, thereby impairing ventilation. Pneumatic antishock garments may also be used initially in the treatment of hypovolemic shock. If shock occurs from hemorrhage, draw blood for possible type and crossmatch and

ensure that the patient has a number 16- to 18-gauge IV access to allow rapid administration of packed RBCs. Insert a Foley catheter to monitor hourly urine output because hourly output reflects the adequacy of fluid replacement.

8. Hypocalcemia may develop in rapidly transfused patients because of the citrate in stored blood. Monitor the patient for sudden symptoms of hypocalcemia (see Chapter 9). As prescribed, administer 10 mL of calcium chloride or gluconate for every 2 units of blood transfused.

9. Hyperkalemia may develop in patients with rapid and massive transfusion from the potassium content of banked blood (20 to 30 mmol/L in blood stored longer than 5 days). Monitor patient for electrocardiogram (ECG) changes associated with hyperkalemia (i.e., tall peaked T wave and widened QRS).

**Ineffective tissue perfusion** related to hypovolemia.

**Desired outcomes:** The patient has adequate perfusion as evidenced by alertness, warm and dry skin, BP within the patient's normal range, HR less than 100 bpm, urinary output more than 0.5 mL/kg/hour for 2 consecutive hours, capillary refill less than 2 seconds, and peripheral pulses greater than 2+ on a 0 to 4+ scale.

1. Monitor for signs of decreased cerebral perfusion: vertigo, syncope, confusion, restlessness, anxiety, agitation, excitability, weakness, nausea, and cool and clammy skin. Alert the physician to worsening symptoms. Document the patient's response to fluid therapy.

2. Protect patients who are confused, dizzy, or weak. Keep side rails up and the bed in its lowest position with the wheels locked. Assist with ambulation in step-down units. Raise the patient to sitting or standing positions slowly. Monitor for indicators of orthostatic hypotension: decreased BP, increased HR, dizziness, and diaphoresis. If symptoms occur, return the patient to a supine position and consult with the physician.

3. To avoid unnecessary vasodilation, treat fevers promptly. Cover the patient with a light blanket to maintain body temperature.

4. Reassure the patient and significant others that sensorium changes improve with therapy.

5. Monitor I&O and alert the physician to a urine output less than 0.5 mL/kg/hour for 2 consecutive hours. Prolonged reduction in renal perfusion may result in ischemic damage to the kidneys and acute renal failure.
6. Evaluate capillary refill, noting whether it is brisk ($<2$ seconds) or delayed ($\geq 2$ seconds). Notify the physician if refill is delayed.
7. Palpate peripheral pulses bilaterally in the arms and legs (radial, brachial, dorsalis pedis, and posterior tibial). Use a Doppler ultrasonic device if unable to palpate pulses. Rate pulses on a 0 to 4+ scale. Notify the physician if pulses are absent or barely palpable. NOTE: Abnormal pulses also may be caused by a local vascular disorder.

For additional nursing diagnoses, see the specific medical disorder, electrolyte imbalance, or acid-base disturbance.

## Patient-Family Teaching Guidelines

Give the patient and significant others verbal and written instructions for the following:
1. Signs and symptoms of hypovolemia
2. Importance of maintaining adequate intake, especially in small children and older adults, who are more likely to dehydrate
3. Medications: name, purpose, dosage, frequency, precautions, and potential side effects

# Hypervolemia

Expansion of ECF volume is termed *hypervolemia*. It occurs whenever there is: (1) chronic stimulus to the kidney to conserve sodium and water; (2) abnormal renal function, with reduced excretion of sodium and water; (3) excessive administration of IV fluids; or (4) interstitial-to-plasma fluid shift. Hypervolemia can lead to heart failure and pulmonary edema (see Chapter 21), especially in a patient with cardiovascular dysfunction. Compensatory mechanisms for hypervolemia include the release of natriuretic peptides (see Chapter 2), leading to increased filtration and excretion of sodium and water by the kidneys and decreased release of aldosterone. Abnormalities in electrolyte homeostasis, acid-base balance, and osmolality often accompany hypervolemia.

## Assessment

1. **Clinical manifestations:** SOB and orthopnea.
2. **Physical assessment:** Edema, weight gain, increased BP (decreased BP as the heart fails), bounding pulses, ascites, crackles (rales), rhonchi, wheezes, tachypnea, distended neck veins, moist skin, tachycardia, and gallop rhythm.
3. **Hemodynamic measurements:** Increased CVP, PAP, and PAWP. MAP is increased unless left heart failure is present.
4. **History and risk factors:**
   - *Retention of sodium and water*
     Heart failure
     Cirrhosis
     Nephrotic syndrome
     Excessive administration of glucocorticosteroids
   - *Abnormal renal function*
     Acute or chronic renal failure with oliguria
   - *Excessive administration of IV fluids*
   - ISF-to-plasma shift
     Remobilization of fluid after treatment of burns and excessive administration of hypertonic solutions (e.g., mannitol, hypertonic saline) or colloid oncotic solutions (e.g., albumin).

## Diagnostic Tests

Laboratory findings are variable and usually nonspecific.
1. **B-type natriuretic peptide (BNP):** Increased. Greater than 100 pg/mL in congestive heart failure.
2. **BUN:** Increased in renal failure.
3. **Hematocrit:** Decreased because of hemodilution.
4. **ABG values:** May reveal hypoxemia (decreased $Pao_2$) and respiratory alkalosis (increased pH and decreased $Paco_2$) in the presence of pulmonary edema.
5. **Serum sodium:** Decreased if hypervolemia occurs as a result of excessive water retention (e.g., in chronic renal failure).
6. **Urinary sodium:** Elevated if the kidney is attempting to excrete excess sodium. Urinary sodium is not elevated in conditions with secondary hyperaldosteronism (e.g., congestive heart failure, cirrhosis, nephrotic syndrome)

because hypervolemia occurs as a result of a chronic stimulus to the release of aldosterone.

7. **Urine specific gravity:** Decreased if the kidney is attempting to excrete excess volume. May be fixed at 1.010 in acute renal failure.

8. **Chest radiograph:** May reveal signs of pulmonary vascular congestion.

## Collaborative Management

The goal of therapy is treatment of the precipitating problem and return of ECF to normal. Treatment may include the following:

1. **Restriction of sodium and water:** Oral, enteral, or parenteral. (Box 6-2 provides a list of foods high in sodium.)

2. **Diuretics:** May be given IV or orally (PO). Loop diuretics (e.g., furosemide) are indicated in severe hypervolemia or renal failure.

3. **Dialysis or continuous renal replacement therapy:** In renal failure or life-threatening fluid overload.

NOTE: Also see the specific discussions on congestive heart failure (Chapter 21), renal failure (Chapter 22), and cirrhosis (Chapter 24).

## Nursing Diagnoses and Interventions

**Excess fluid volume** related to excessive fluid or sodium intake or compromised regulatory mechanism.

---

### Box 6-2    Foods High in Sodium

- Bouillon
- Celery
- Cheeses
- Dried fruits
- Frozen, canned, or packaged foods
- Ketchup
- Monosodium glutamate (MSG)
- Mustard
- Olives
- Pickles
- Preserved meat
- Salad dressings and prepared sauces
- Sauerkraut
- Snack foods (e.g., crackers, chips, pretzels)
- Soy sauce

**Desired outcomes:** The patient is normovolemic as evidenced by adequate urinary output of more than 0.5 mL/kg/hour, specific gravity of approximately 1.010 to 1.020, stable weights, and absence of edema. BP is within the patient's normal range, CVP is 2 to 6 mm Hg, and HR is 60 to 100 bpm. In addition, for critical care patients, PAP is 20 to 30/8 to 15 mm Hg, MAP is 70 to 105 mm Hg, and CO is 4 to 7 L/minute.

1. Monitor I&O hourly. Except for oliguric renal failure, urine output should be more than 0.5 mL/kg/hour. Measure urine specific gravity every shift. If the patient is undergoing diuretic therapy, specific gravity should be less than 1.010 to 1.020.

2. Observe for and document presence of edema: pretibial, sacral, and periorbital. Rate pitting on a 1 to 4 scale (Figure 6-2).

3. Weigh the patient daily. Daily weights are the single most important indicator of fluid status. For example, a 2-kg acute weight gain is indicative of a 2-L fluid gain. Weigh the patient at the same time each day (preferably before breakfast) on a balanced scale, with the patient wearing approximately the same clothing. Document the type of scale used (e.g., standing, bed, chair).

4. Obtain an accurate dietary history and limit sodium intake as prescribed by the physician (see Box 6-2). Consider the use of salt substitutes. NOTE: Salt substitutes contain potassium and may be contraindicated in patients with renal failure or receiving potassium-sparing diuretics (e.g., spironolactone, triamterene). Incorporate cultural considerations when providing dietary counseling.

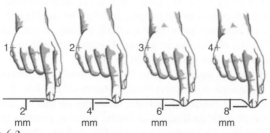

Figure 6-2
Assessment of pitting edema: 1+, 2+, 3+, and 4+.

5. Limit fluids as prescribed. Offer a portion of allotted fluids as ice chips to minimize the patient's thirst. Teach the patient and significant others the importance of fluid restriction and how to measure fluid volume.

6. Provide oral hygiene at frequent intervals to keep oral mucous membranes moist and intact.

7. Document the patient's response to diuretic therapy (e.g., increased urine output, decreased CVP/PAP, decreased adventitious breath sounds, decreased edema). Many diuretics (e.g., furosemide, thiazides) cause hypokalemia. Observe for indicators of hypokalemia: muscle weakness, dysrhythmias (especially premature ventricular contractions [PVCs] and ECG changes [e.g., flattened T wave, presence of U waves]; see p. 114). Potassium-sparing diuretics (e.g., spironolactone, triamterene) may cause hyperkalemia; indicators include weakness and ECG changes (e.g., peaked T wave, prolonged PR interval, widened QRS; see p. 114). Consult the physician for significant findings.

8. Observe for physical indicators of overcorrection and dangerous volume depletion from therapy: vertigo, weakness, syncope, thirst, confusion, poor skin turgor, flat neck veins, and acute weight loss. Monitor VS and hemodynamic parameters for signs of volume depletion occurring with therapy: decreased BP, CVP, PAP, MAP, and CO and increased HR. Consult the physician for abnormal trends.

**Gas exchange, impaired** (or risk for) related to alveolar-capillary membrane changes from pulmonary vascular congestion occurring with ECF expansion.

**Desired outcomes:** The patient has adequate gas exchange as evidenced by a resting rate of 20 or fewer breaths/minute, HR 100 or fewer breaths per minute, and Pao$_2$ 80 mm Hg or higher. The patient does not exhibit crackles, gallops, or other clinical indicators of pulmonary edema. For patients in critical care, PAP is less than or equal to 30/15 mm Hg.

1. Acute pulmonary edema is a potentially life-threatening complication of hypervolemia. Monitor the patient for indicators of pulmonary edema, including air hunger, anxiety, cough with production of frothy sputum, crackles (rales), rhonchi, tachypnea, tachycardia, gallop rhythm, and

elevation of PAP and pulmonary artery wedge pressure (PAWP). Administer loop diuretics as prescribed to induce peripheral vasodilation and decreased venous return.

2. Monitor ABGs for evidence of hypoxemia (decreased $Pao_2$) and respiratory alkalosis (increased pH and decreased $Paco_2$); monitor pulse oximetry for decreased oxygen saturation. Administer oxygen as prescribed. Increased oxygen requirements may indicate increasing pulmonary vascular congestion.

3. Keep the patient in semi-Fowler's position or in a position of comfort to minimize dyspnea. Avoid restrictive clothing.

**Skin integrity, risk for impaired** related to edema from fluid volume excess.

**Desired outcome:** The patient's skin and tissue remain intact.

1. Assess and document circulation to extremities at least every shift. Note color, temperature, capillary refill, and peripheral pulses. Determine whether capillary refill is brisk ($< 2$ seconds) or delayed (2 seconds). Palpate peripheral pulses bilaterally in the arms and legs (radial, brachial, dorsalis pedis, and posterior tibial). Use Doppler device if unable to palpate pulses. Consult with the physician if capillary refill is delayed or pulses are absent.

2. Turn and reposition the patient at least every 2 hours to minimize tissue pressure.

3. Check tissue areas at risk with each position change (e.g., heels, sacrum, and other areas over bony prominences).

4. Use pressure-relief mattresses as indicated.

5. Support the arms and hands on pillows and elevate the legs to decrease dependent edema (unless pulmonary edema or heart failure is present).

6. Treat pressure ulcers with occlusive dressings (e.g., Duoderm, Op-Site, Tegaderm) per unit protocol. Notify the physician of the presence of sores, ulcers, or areas of tissue breakdown in patients who are at increased risk for infection (e.g., individuals with diabetes or renal failure, those with immunosuppression).

7. Consult a skin/wound care nurse specialist, as available, for advanced tissue breakdown or any alteration in tissue

integrity in high-risk patients (e.g., those at an advanced age or debilitated).

## Patient-Family Teaching Guidelines

Give the patient and significant others verbal and written instructions for the following:

1. Signs and symptoms of hypervolemia.
2. Symptoms that necessitate physician notification after hospital discharge: SOB, chest pain, and new pulse irregularity.
3. Low-sodium diet, if prescribed; use of a salt substitute; avoidance of foods that are high in sodium (see Box 6-2); and maintenance of a high-potassium diet or need for potassium supplement if on loop or thiazide-type diuretics (see Box 8-1).
4. Medications: name, purpose, dosage, frequency, precautions, and potential side effects; signs and symptoms of hypokalemia if the patient is taking diuretics.
5. Importance of fluid restriction if hypervolemia continues.
6. Importance of daily weights and when to consult a physician for weight gain (e.g., call for weight gain of > 2 pounds [lbs]/day).
7. Patient should take once-daily doses of diuretics in the morning to minimize night voiding. With twice a day dosing, the second dose should be no later than 4 PM.
8. If patient is on diuretics, the patient should avoid prolonged standing and rise slowly from lying or sitting to prevent postural hypotension.

## Edema Formation

Edema occurs as a result of expansion of the ISF volume and is defined as a palpable swelling of the interstitial space that is either localized (e.g., thrombophlebitis with venous obstruction) or generalized (e.g., cardiac failure). Severe generalized edema is termed *anasarca*. Edema may develop any time an alteration in capillary hemodynamics favors either increased formation or decreased removal of ISF (Figure 6-3). Increased capillary hydrostatic pressure from volume expansion or venous obstruction, or increased capillary permeability owing to burns, allergy, or infection, causes an increase in ISF volume.

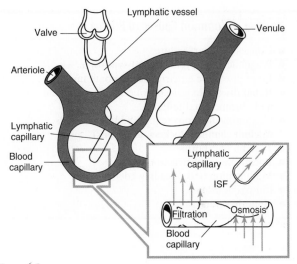

Figure 6-3
Capillary diagram.

Decreased removal of ISF occurs with an obstruction to lymphatic outflow or a decrease in plasma oncotic pressure (remember that the plasma proteins help hold the vascular volume in the vascular space). Furthermore, retention of sodium and water by the kidneys enhances and maintains generalized edema. This may result from a decreased ability to excrete sodium and water (overflow) as in renal failure or from an increased stimulus to conserve sodium and water (underfilling). In heart failure, for example, impaired cardiac function leads to a reduction in CO with a drop in effective circulating volume, which in turn stimulates the kidneys to conserve sodium and water via the renin-angiotensin system and water via increased ADH. As the patient with heart failure retains volume, the venous circuit expands, capillary hydrostatic pressure increases, and edema is formed. The edema seen in nephrotic syndrome and hepatic cirrhosis (ascites; see Chapter 24) is the result of both underfilling and overflow. (Box 6-3 lists the most common causes of edema.)

---

### Box 6-3    Common Causes of Edema

- Congestive heart failure
- Pregnancy and premenstrual syndrome
- Liver disease (e.g., cirrhosis, hypoalbuminemia)
- Renal disease (e.g., nephrotic syndrome, acute and chronic renal failure)
- Certain medications (e.g., NSAIDs, steroids, calcium channel blockers, estrogens)
- Trauma and burns
- Local venous obstruction
- Malnutrition and refeeding edema
- Idiopathic edema
- Hypothyroidism

---

## Assessment

Generalized edema usually is most evident in dependent areas. The ambulatory patient exhibits pretibial or ankle edema, whereas the patient restricted to bed exhibits sacral edema. Generalized edema also may present around the eyes (periorbital) or in the scrotal sac because of the low tissue pressures in these areas. To identify sacral edema, press the index finger firmly into the sacral tissue and maintain pressure for several seconds. If a pit remains after the finger has been withdrawn, edema is present. Pitting also may be assessed over the tibia or ankle. Pitting should be rated according to severity (see Figure 6-2). (See Chapter 21 for a discussion of pulmonary edema.)

## Collaborative Management

1. **Treatment of the primary problem (e.g., digitalis for patients with congestive heart failure).**
2. **Mobilization of edema (e.g., with bed rest and supportive hose).**
3. **Dietary restriction of sodium:** In addition, hidden sodium sources (e.g., medications) should be avoided.
4. **Diuretic therapy:** See the subsequent section.

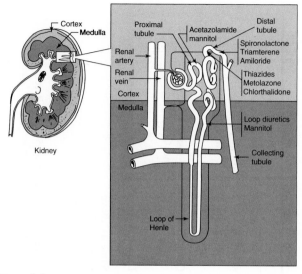

Figure 6-4
Sites of diuretic action.

5. **Dialysis or continuous renal replacement therapy (e.g., for renal failure or life-threatening fluid overload).**
6. **Abdominal paracentesis (e.g., for the treatment of severe ascites that adversely affects cardiopulmonary functioning).**

## Diuretic Therapy

Diuretics reduce edema by inhibiting the resorption of sodium, and therefore water, by the kidneys. Diuretics also may induce the loss of other important electrolytes and alter the acid-base balance. Although retention of sodium and water by the kidneys is an important component in the development of edema, not all edematous states require treatment with diuretics. Reduction in the effective circulating volume and alterations in electrolyte balance caused by diuretics may be detrimental. Patients with hepatic cirrhosis, for example, may develop hepatic coma or hepatorenal syndrome related to

Table 6-7   Diuretic action

| Diuretic (by primary site of action) | Potency | Characteristic of Diuresis |
|---|---|---|
| **Proximal Tubule** | | |
| Acetazolamide (Diamox)* | Weak | $NaHCO_3$ diuresis with loss of additional $Na^+$, $Cl^-$, and phosphorus |
| **Proximal Tubule and Loop** | | |
| Mannitol[†] | Moderate | Osmotic diuresis with loss of water in excess of $Na^+$ and $Cl^-$ |
| **Loop of Henle** | | |
| Furosemide (Lasix)[‡] | Strong | Large diuresis (may affect 25% of filtered load of sodium) with loss of $Na^+$, $Cl^-$, and $K^+$ |
| Ethacrynic acid (Edecrin)[‡] | Strong | Same as above |
| Bumetanide (Bumex) | Strong | Same as above |
| Torsemide (Demadex)[‡] | Strong | Same as above |
| **Early Distal Tubule** | | |
| Thiazides (Diuril, Hydrodiuril, Esidrix)[§] | Moderate | Diuresis affecting up to 5% of filtered load of sodium, with loss of $Cl^-$ and $K^+$ |
| Metolazone (Zaroxolyn)[§] | Moderate | Same as above |
| Chlorthalidone (Hygroton)[§] | Moderate | Same as above |
| Indanamide (Lozol)[‖] | Moderate | Same as above |

Late Distal Tubule—Potassium-
Sparing Diuretics

| | | |
|---|---|---|
| Spironolactone (Aldactone)¶ | Weak | Blocks action of aldosterone, with loss of $Na^+$ and $Cl^-$ but not $K^+$ |
| Triamterene (Dyrenium)¶ | Weak | Weak diuresis with loss of $Na^+$ and $Cl^-$ but not $K^+$; does not depend on presence of aldosterone |
| Amiloride (Midamor)¶ | Weak | Same as triamterene |

Clinical indications and nursing considerations:

*May be used in the treatment of metabolic alkalosis. It is most commonly used to treat glaucoma because it decreases the formation of aqueous humor. It is contraindicated in patients with acidosis.

†May cause hyperosmolality and circulatory overload because of the osmotic shift of fluid out of the cells and into the interstitium and intravascular space. Use with caution in patients with decreased cardiac function. The patient should be monitored for signs of circulatory overload (e.g., crackles, SOB, tachycardia). It may be used in the treatment of early acute renal failure, elevated intracranial pressure, and cerebral edema.

‡Used to treat edema of congestive heart failure and advanced renal failure. It may be used alone or in combination with mannitol or dopamine to reverse early acute renal failure. It is effective in the treatment of acute pulmonary edema because of its diuretic and direct venous vasodilatory actions. It should not be given rapidly by IV because of the risk of ototoxicity (tinnitus or hearing loss). Stop the infusion and notify the physician if the patient has ringing in the ears. The patient should be monitored for hypokalemia (see Chapter 8) and volume depletion (see this chapter).

§Often used to treat hypertension because of diuretic action and antihypertensive effect, which is unrelated to diuretic action. This group of diuretics has the most nondiuresis-related side effects (e.g., decreased release of insulin, hyperlipidemia, skin rashes). The patient should be monitored for hypokalemia (see Chapter 8), hyperglycemia, and volume depletion (see this chapter). These diuretics also may cause hyperuricemia and hypercalcemia (see Chapter 9).

‖Similar to the thiazides in action and use but does not cause hyperlipidemia or hyperglycemia.

¶May be combined with thiazide diuretics for increased diuretic action and less hypokalemia. These diuretics may cause hyperkalemia (see Chapter 8). Concurrent use of other potassium-sparing diuretics or salt substitutes should be avoided.

diuretic-induced hypokalemia and rapid fluid removal. Most patients with edema, however, may benefit from the careful use of diuretics.

The quantity and characteristics of the diuresis vary depending on the type of diuretic and its site of action within the renal tubule (Figure 6-4 and Table 6-7). Although some complications of diuretic therapy are common to all or most diuretics (see the subsequent discussion), the specifics of nursing care depend on the type of diuretic the patient is receiving (see Table 6-7).

## Complications of Diuretic Therapy

1. **Volume abnormalities:** Volume depletion caused by over-diuresis. May develop as a result of excessive dose, improved compliance with existing dose, reduction in dietary sodium, or improvement in underlying condition. Monitor patients for signs of fluid volume deficit: dizziness, weakness, fatigue, and postural hypotension.

2. **Electrolyte disturbances:**
   - *Hypokalemia:* Occurs as a result of increased secretion and excretion of potassium by the kidneys. It may occur with all the diuretics except for those that work in the late distal tubule. Hypokalemia can be avoided by giving a potassium-sparing diuretic (see Table 6-7) or a potassium supplement. Monitor patients for indicators of hypokalemia: fatigue, muscle weakness, leg cramps, and irregular pulse.
   - *Hyperkalemia:* Occurs because of decreased secretion and excretion of potassium by the kidneys. It may occur with diuretics that work in the late distal tubule (see Table 6-7). The potassium-sparing diuretics should not be given to patients with decreased renal function (because of the increased risk of hyperkalemia) or those receiving a potassium supplement. Concomitant use of certain medications, such as nonsteroidal antiinflammatory drugs (NSAIDs), angiotensin-converting enzyme (ACE) inhibitors, and tacrolimus, increase the risk of hyperkalemia. Monitor patients for indicators of hyperkalemia: irritability, anxiety, abdominal cramping, muscle weakness (especially in the lower extremities), and ECG changes. (See Chapter 8 for additional information.)

- *Hyponatremia:* Occurs because of a decreased ability to excrete solute free water and increased release of ADH. It is most common with the thiazide-type diuretics. Monitor patients for indicators of hyponatremia: nausea, vomiting, lethargy, and confusion.

- *Hypomagnesemia:* Occurs because of decreased resorption and increased excretion of magnesium by the kidneys. This may occur with the loop and thiazide-type diuretics and contributes to the development of hypokalemia. Potassium-sparing diuretics may be used to prevent urinary magnesium wasting. Monitor patients for indicators of hypomagnesemia: confusion, cramps, and dysrhythmias. Unfortunately, most magnesium loss occurs from the intracellular space, and serum values may remain deceptively normal.

- *Hypercalcemia:* May occur with the thiazide diuretics because of decreased urinary excretion of calcium.

3. **Acid-base disturbances:**

- *Metabolic alkalosis:* May be caused by the loop and thiazide-type diuretics because of increased secretion and excretion of hydrogen by the kidneys and contraction of the ECF around the existing bicarbonate *(contraction alkalosis)*. Hypokalemia, if present, perpetuates alkalosis. Monitor patients for indicators of metabolic alkalosis: muscular weakness, dysrhythmias, apathy, and confusion.

- *Metabolic acidosis:* May occur with acetazolamide therapy as a result of increased loss of bicarbonate in the urine. Monitor patients for indicators of metabolic acidosis: tachypnea, fatigue, and confusion. Metabolic acidosis may also occur with potassium-sparing diuretics.

4. **Other metabolic complications:**

- *Azotemia:* Increased retention of metabolic wastes (e.g., urea, creatinine) resulting from a reduction in effective circulating volume with decreased perfusion of the kidneys and decreased excretion of metabolic wastes. Consult with the physician for changes in a patient's BUN and serum creatinine levels.

- *Hyperuricemia:* Occurs as a result of increased resorption and decreased excretion of uric acid by the kidneys. Consult with the physician regarding patient symptoms of gout-type pain. This condition usually is problematic only in patients with preexisting gout.

- *Hyperlipidemia and hyperglycemia:* May occur with the use of thiazide and (occasionally) loop diuretics. This is of greatest concern in patients with diabetes.

5. **Toxic complications:**

- *Ototoxicity:* The loop diuretics may cause tinnitus or hearing loss especially with rapid administration of large parenteral doses.

## Intravenous Fluid Therapy

The goals of IV fluid therapy are to maintain or restore normal fluid volume and electrolyte balance and to provide a means of administering medications quickly and efficiently. An additional concern is that of nutrition. Unfortunately, routine IV fluids (e.g., 5% dextrose solutions) contain only enough carbohydrates to minimize tissue breakdown and starvation. They do not provide adequate calories and essential amino acids needed for tissue synthesis. For example, 5% dextrose solutions supply only 170 to 200 calories per liter, whereas the average patient on bed rest requires a minimum of 1500 calories a day. Patients should not be maintained solely on 5% dextrose solutions for longer than a few days. (See Chapter 26 for a discussion of nutritional therapies and total parenteral nutrition [TPN].)

The type of IV fluid prescribed for volume replacement or maintenance depends on several factors, including the type of fluid lost and the patient's nutritional needs, serum electrolytes, serum osmolality, and acid-base balance. (Figure 6-5 provides a comparison of lactated Ringer's solution, 0.9% NaCl, and 0.45% NaCl to ECF.)

### Commonly Prescribed Intravenous Fluids

Intravenous fluids are divided into two major categories: crystalloids and colloids. *Crystalloid solutions* contain only electrolytes and glucose, substances that are not restricted to the intravascular space. Therefore these solutions expand the entire extracellular space. Depending on their sodium content, crystalloids also may expand the ICF volume. Isotonic NaCl (0.9%) and Ringer's solution expand only the ECF, whereas

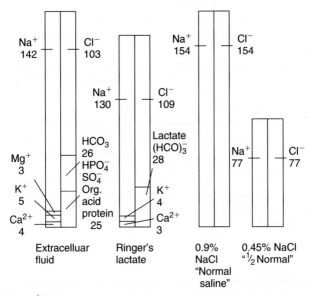

Figure 6-5
Comparison of extracellular fluid and three common IV
solutions (29 mmol/L).

hypotonic NaCl solutions and dextrose and water solutions
expand all fluid compartments. Crystalloids are typically
classified according to the osmolarity (tonicity) of the solution.
Isotonic solutions have an osmolarity similar to plasma,
hypotonic solutions have an osmolarity significantly less than
plasma, and hypertonic solutions have an osmolarity significantly greater than plasma. Because of the risk of RBC
hemolysis, there is a limit to how hypotonic a fluid may be
and still be safely administered IV. Pure water and hypotonic
saline solutions such as 0.225% NaCl require the addition of
5% dextrose to allow safe administration. For the clinician
administering IV fluids, it is important to consider the "true"
tonicity of the solution. Although both normal saline (0.9%
NaCl) and 5% dextrose in water ($D_5W$) are considered isotonic (osmolarity similar to plasma) before administration,
$D_5W$ is in fact a hypotonic fluid once it has been administered
and the dextrose has been metabolized. Advantages of

crystalloids are that they are relatively inexpensive and non-allergenic. (Table 6-3 compares commonly prescribed crystalloid solutions.)

*Colloid solutions* contain cells, proteins, or synthetic macromolecules that do not readily cross the capillary membrane. These solutions remain within the vascular space and, depending on their concentration, may cause an osmotic shift of fluids from the interstitium into the intravascular space. Disadvantages of colloids can include increased cost, risk of allergic reactions, and clotting abnormalities. (Table 6-4 compares commonly prescribed colloid solutions.) Blood is the most commonly administered colloid. (Box 6-4 provides information on nursing management of transfusion reactions; Table 6-8 lists common causes of blood transfusion reactions.)

---

### Box 6-4    When a Transfusion Reaction Occurs

1. STOP THE TRANSFUSION.
2. Keep the IV line open with 0.9% normal saline solution.
3. Report the reaction to both the transfusion service and attending physician immediately.
4. Do a clerical check of identifying tags and numbers at the bedside.
5. Treat the symptoms per physician's order, and monitor vital signs.
6. Send the blood bag with the attached administration set and labels to the transfusion service.
7. Collect blood and urine samples and send them to the laboratory.*
8. Document thoroughly on a transfusion reaction form and the patient's chart.

From National Blood Resource Education Programs: *Transfusion therapy guidelines for nurses,* NIH Publication No. 90-2668a, 1990, National Institutes of Health.

*Check with the transfusion service to determine the specific blood and urine samples needed to evaluate reactions.

| Reaction | Cause | Clinical Manifestations | Management | Prevention |
|---|---|---|---|---|
| Acute hemolytic | Infusion of ABO-incompatible whole blood, RBCs, or components containing 10 mL or more of RBCs. Antibodies in recipient's plasma attach to antigens on transfused RBCs, causing RBC destruction. | Chills, fever, low back pain, flushing, tachycardia, tachypnea, hypotension, vascular collapse, hemoglobinuria, acute renal failure, bleeding, shock, cardiac arrest, death | Treat shock, if present. Draw blood samples for serologic testing slowly to avoid hemolysis from procedure. Send urine specimen to laboratory. Maintain BP with IV colloid solutions. Give diuretics as prescribed to maintain urine flow. Insert indwelling catheter or measure voided amounts to monitor hourly urine output. Dialysis may be necessary if renal failure occurs. | Meticulously verify and document patient identification from sample collection to component infusion. |

*Continued*

Table 6-8   Acute transfusion reactions—cont'd

| Reaction | Cause | Clinical Manifestations | Management | Prevention |
|---|---|---|---|---|
| | | | Do not transfuse additional **RBC-containing components** until transfusion service has provided newly crossmatched units. | |
| Febrile, non-hemolytic (most common) | Sensitization to donor WBCs, platelets or plasma proteins. | Sudden chills and fever (rise in temperature of greater than 1° C), headache, flushing, anxiety, muscle pain | Give antipyretics as prescribed; avoid aspirin in thrombocytopenic patients. **Do not restart transfusion.** | Consider leukocyte-poor blood products (filtered, washed, or frozen). |
| Mild allergic | Sensitivity to foreign plasma proteins. | Flushing, itching, urticaria (hives) | Give antihistamines as directed. If symptoms are mild and transient, transfusion may be | Treat prophylactically with antihistamines. |

| Anaphylactic | Infusion of IgA proteins to IgA-deficient recipient who has developed IgA antibodies. | Anxiety, urticaria, and wheezing, progressing to cyanosis, shock, and possible cardiac arrest | ...sion if fever or pulmonary symptoms develop. Initiate CPR, if indicated. Have epinephrine ready for injection (0.4 mL of 1:1000 solution subcutaneously or 0.1 mL of 1:1000 solution diluted to 10 mL with saline solution for IV use). **Do not restart transfusion.** | Transfuse extensively washed RBC products from which all plasma has been removed. Alternatively, use blood from IgA-deficient donor. |

*Continued*

Table 6-8   Acute transfusion reactions—cont'd

| Reaction | Cause | Clinical Manifestations | Management | Prevention |
|---|---|---|---|---|
| Circulatory overload | Fluid administered faster than circulation can accommodate. | Cough, dyspnea, pulmonary congestion (rales), headache, hypertension, tachycardia, distended neck veins | Place patient upright with feet in dependent position. Administer prescribed diuretics, oxygen, and morphine. Phlebotomy may be indicated. | Adjust transfusion volume and flow rate based on patient's size and clinical status. Have transfusion service divide each unit into smaller aliquots for better spacing of fluid input. |
| Sepsis | Transfusion of contaminated blood components. | Rapid onset of chills, high fever, vomiting, diarrhea, and marked hypotension and shock | Obtain culture of patient's blood and send bag with remaining blood to transfusion service for further study. Treat septicemia as directed (e.g., with antibiotics, IV fluids, vasopressors, steroids). | Collect, process, store, and transfuse blood products according to blood banking standards and infuse them within 4 hours of starting time. |

From National Blood Resource Education Programs: *Transfusion therapy guidelines for nurses,* NIH Publication No. 90-2668a, 1990, National Institutes of Health.
*CPR,* Cardiopulmonary resuscitation; *IgA,* immunoglobulin A.

# Disorders of Sodium Balance

7

Sodium plays a vital role in the maintenance of concentration and volume of extracellular fluid (ECF). It is the main cation of ECF and the major determinant of ECF osmolality. In normal conditions, ECF osmolality can be estimated by doubling the serum sodium value. Sodium imbalances are usually associated with parallel changes in osmolality. Sodium also is important in maintaining irritability and conduction of nerve and muscle tissue, and it assists with the regulation of acid-base balance.

## Sodium Changes

The average daily intake of sodium far exceeds the body's normal daily requirements. The kidneys are responsible for excreting the excess and are capable of conserving sodium avidly during periods of extreme sodium restriction. The hormones angiotensin II, aldosterone, and the natriuretic peptides are the primary regulators of renal sodium excretion. Both angiotensin II and aldosterone enhance renal sodium conservation. The major stimulus to the release of angiotensin II is a low ECF volume; aldosterone, in turn, is released in response to increased angiotensin II. In contrast, the natriuretic peptides increase renal excretion of sodium in response to ECF volume expansion.

Sodium concentration (the relationship between sodium and water in the plasma) is maintained via regulation of water intake and excretion. If serum sodium is elevated (hypernatremia), serum osmolality increases, stimulating the thirst center and causing an increased release of antidiuretic hormone (ADH) by the posterior pituitary gland. ADH acts on the kidneys to conserve water. The combination of an increased water intake and renal water conservation helps restore the normal sodium level. Conversely, when the serum sodium concentration is decreased (hyponatremia), the kidneys respond by excreting excess water. Thus changes in serum sodium levels typically reflect changes in water balance. Gains or losses of total body sodium are not necessarily reflected by the serum sodium level but rather by the total volume of body fluid. Normal serum sodium levels are 135 to 145 milliequivalents/liter (mmol/L).

## Hyponatremia

Hyponatremia (serum sodium < 135 mmol/L) can occur because of a net gain of water or loss of sodium-rich fluids that are replaced by water. The most important defense against the development of hyponatremia is renal excretion of sodium-free water; thus hyponatremia is most likely to develop with a physiologic stimulus to conserve water. Hyponatremia is typically associated with hypoosmolality and is the most common electrolyte imbalance in hospitalized patients. Clinical indicators and treatment depend on the rapidity of onset and cause of hyponatremia and on whether it is associated with a normal, decreased, or increased ECF volume.

The symptoms of hyponatremia are largely the result of an intracellular shift of water that occurs with hyponatremia-induced hypoosmolality. Because of the fixed volume of the skull, symptoms of acute hyponatremia occur as a result of cerebral edema and increased intracranial pressure. However, the brain possesses the ability to adapt over time to hypoosmolality by reducing intracellular solutes and thus limiting the increase in cerebral water. Thus at a given sodium level, chronic hyponatremia is associated with less symptoms than acute hyponatremia. This important adaptive mechanism can cause a dangerously rapid loss of cerebral water if hyponatremia is corrected too rapidly. (For more information, see pp. 24-25.)

### Assessment

1. **Clinical manifestations:**
   NOTE: Neurologic symptoms usually do not occur until the serum sodium level has dropped to approximately 120 to 125 mmol/L or less. Seizures, coma, and permanent neurologic damage may occur when the plasma sodium level is less than 115 mmol/L. Patients at increased risk for neurologic

complications of hyponatremia include children, premeno-
pausal women, polydipsic psychiatric patients, older adult
patients on thiazide diuretics, and hypoxic patients.

- *Hyponatremia with decreased ECF volume:* Irritability,
  apprehension, dizziness, personality changes, postural
  hypotension, dry mucous membranes, cold and clammy
  skin, tremors, seizures, and coma.
- *Hyponatremia with normal or increased ECF volume:*
  Headache, lassitude, apathy, confusion, weakness, edema,
  weight gain, elevated blood pressure (BP), muscle cramps,
  convulsions, and coma.

2. **Hemodynamic measurements:**
- *Decreased ECF volume:* Evidence of hypovolemia, including decreased central venous pressure (CVP), pulmonary
  artery pressure (PAP), cardiac output (CO), mean arterial
  pressure (MAP), and increased systemic vascular resistance (SVR).
- *Increased ECF volume:* Evidence of hypervolemia, including increased CVP, PAP, and MAP.

3. **History and risk factors:**
- *Decreased ECF volume*
  Gastrointestinal (GI) losses: Diarrhea, vomiting, fistulas,
    and nasogastric (NG) suction
  Renal losses: Diuretics, salt wasting kidney disease,
    adrenal insufficiency, and cerebral salt wasting (renal
    salt wasting associated with cerebral injury)
  Skin losses: Burns and wound drainage
- *Normal/increased ECF volume*
  Syndrome of inappropriate secretion of antidiuretic
    hormone (SIADH): Excessive production of ADH
    (see Chapter 20)
  Edematous states: Congestive heart failure, cirrhosis, and
    nephrotic syndrome
  Excessive administration of hypotonic intravenous (IV)
    fluids
  Oliguric renal failure
  Primary psychogenic polydipsia
- *Hyperglycemia:* With hyperglycemia, the osmotic action
  of the elevated glucose causes a shift of water out of
  the cells and into the ECF, thus diluting the existing
  sodium. For every 100 milligrams/deciliter (mg/dL) the

glucose is elevated, sodium is diluted by 1.6 mmol/L. Hyponatremia in this situation is associated with increased osmolality related to the increased glucose.

■ *Pseudohyponatremia:* Hyperlipidemia and hyperproteinemia may cause a pseudohyponatremia. Markedly elevated plasma lipids or proteins reduce the total percentage of water in plasma. The sodium/water ratio of the plasma does not change, but the plasma sodium level is reduced because of a reduction in plasma water. This type of pseudohyponatremia is now rare because of a change in the method used by most clinical laboratories to measure serum sodium levels.

NOTE: Older adults are at increased risk for hyponatremia because of decreased renal conservation of sodium and decreased ability to excrete free water that occurs with aging. As a population they are more likely to be on medications that either decrease the ability to excrete free water or increase renal sodium loss.

## Diagnostic Tests

1. **Serum sodium:** Is less than 135 mmol/L.
2. **Serum osmolality:** Decreased, except in cases of pseudohyponatremia (e.g., hyperglycemia), azotemia, or ingestion of toxins that increase osmolality (e.g., ethanol, methanol).
3. **Urine specific gravity:** Decreased because of the kidneys' attempt to excrete excess water. In patients with SIADH, the urine is inappropriately concentrated.
4. **Urine sodium:** Decreased (usually < 20 mmol/L), except in SIADH and adrenal insufficiency.

## Collaborative Management

The immediate goal of therapy is the correction of acute symptoms, the gradual return of sodium to a normal level, and, if necessary, the restoration of normal ECF volume. Acute symptomatic hyponatremia requires more aggressive treatment than does chronic asymptomatic hyponatremia, even when the plasma sodium level is the same. Treatment must be individualized, with both the severity of the hyponatremia and the rate at which it developed taken into account. Permanent neurologic damage may occur in patients with acu4te symptomatic hyponatremia as the result of a failure to adequately treat hyponatremic encephalopathy but also because of overly rapid or aggressive treatment of chronic hyponatremia. The serum sodium level should not be increased greater than 12 mmol/L in 24 hours in either case.

## Hyponatremia with Reduced Extracellular Fluid Volume

1. **Replacement of sodium and fluid losses:** Adequate replacement of fluid volume is essential to turn off the physiologic stimulus to ADH release and to enable the kidneys to restore the balance between sodium and water.
2. **Replacement of other electrolyte losses:** For example, potassium or bicarbonate.
3. **IV hypertonic saline solution:** If serum sodium is dangerously low or the patient is very symptomatic. Used only until the patient's neurologic condition improves or a safe sodium level has been attained. The goal is to give enough 3% sodium chloride (NaCl) to correct symptoms, not to return the sodium level to normal. A loop diuretic may be prescribed with the hypertonic saline solution to increase water excretion and avoid ECF fluid overload.

## Hyponatremia with Expanded Extracellular Fluid Volume

1. **Removal or treatment of the underlying cause:** For example, treatment of SIADH.
2. **Loop diuretic:** Thiazide diuretics should be avoided.
3. **Water restriction:** Restricting fluid intake to 1000 milliliters (mL)/day establishes negative water balance and increases plasma sodium levels in most adults.

NOTE: Too-rapid correction of chronic hyponatremia (lasting > 24 to 48 hours) may result in irreversible neurologic damage and death as a result of osmotic demyelination (central pontine myelinolysis).

## Nursing Diagnoses and Interventions

**Deficient fluid volume** related to abnormal fluid loss; **excess fluid volume** related to excessive intake of hypotonic solutions or increased retention of water.

**Desired outcomes:** The patient is normovolemic as evidenced by a heart rate (HR) of 60 to 100 beats per minute (bpm), respiratory rate (RR) 12 to 20 breaths/minute, BP within the patient's normal range, and CVP 2 to 6 millimeters of mercury (mm Hg). For critical care patients, PAP is 20 to 30/8 to 15 mm Hg.

1. If the patient is receiving hypertonic saline solution, assess carefully for signs of intravascular fluid overload: tachypnea, tachycardia, shortness of breath (SOB), crackles, rhonchi, increased CVP, increased PAP, gallop rhythm, and increased BP. If given too rapidly, hypertonic saline solution may cause crenation (shriveling) of the red blood cells (RBCs) in addition to causing an osmotic shift of fluid into the vascular space. Consult with the physician once neurologic symptoms are relieved in the patient treated with 3% NaCl. The goal of treatment with hypertonic saline solution is to relieve cerebral edema, not to raise the plasma sodium level to normal.

2. For other interventions, see pp. 73 and 76-78 for deficient fluid volume and pp. 80-84 for excess fluid volume.

**Ineffective protection** related to neurosensory alterations from a serum sodium level less than 120 to 125 mmol/L or too-rapid correction of hyponatremia.

**Desired outcome:** The patient verbalizes orientation to person, place, and time and does not exhibit signs of physical injury caused by altered sensorium. The serum sodium level increases no greater than 24 mmol/L in the 48 hours after treatment is initiated.

1. Assess and document level of consciousness (LOC), orientation, and neurologic status with each vital sign (VS) check. Reorient the patient as necessary. Consult the physician for significant changes.

2. Inform the patient and significant others that altered sensorium is temporary and improves with treatment.

3. Keep the side rails up and the bed in its lowest position, with the wheels locked.

4. Use reality therapy such as clocks, calendars, and familiar objects; keep these items at the bedside within the patient's visual field.

5. If seizures are expected, pad side rails and keep an appropriate-size airway at the bedside.

6. Monitor serum sodium levels closely. Permanent neurologic damage may occur with untreated severely symptomatic hyponatremia as a result of cerebral edema. However, overly aggressive or inappropriate treatment can also cause permanent neurologic damage from osmotic demyelination syndrome. Initially plasma sodium levels should not increase at a rate greater than 0.5 to 1 mmol/L/hour in patients being treated with hypertonic NaCl for acute symptomatic hyponatremia. After correction of symptoms, the rate of increase should not be greater than 0.5 mmol/L/hour. Levels should not increase at an average rate of greater than 0.5 mmol/L/hour in patients without symptoms. Caution should be used in treating chronic asymptomatic patients. The overall increase during the first 24 hours of treatment should not exceed 12 mmol/L, or 24 mmol/L in 48 hours.

## Patient-Family Teaching Guidelines

Give the patient and significant others verbal and written instructions for the following:

1. Medications: name, purpose, dosage, frequency, precautions, and potential side effects. Teach signs and symptoms of hypokalemia if the patient is taking diuretics and provide examples of foods that are high in potassium (see Box 8-1).
2. Fluid restriction, if prescribed. Teach the patient that a portion of fluid allotment can be taken as ice or Popsicles to minimize thirst.
3. Signs and symptoms of hypovolemia if hypernatremia is related to abnormal fluid losses.

## Hypernatremia

Hypernatremia (serum sodium level > 145 mmol/L) may occur with water loss, water deprivation, or (rarely) sodium gain. Because the primary defense against hypernatremia is increased thirst, hypernatremia typically occurs in the setting of decreased water intake (e.g., altered thirst, restricted access to water). The other physiologic protection from hypernatremia is the excretion of maximally concentrated urine through increased production of ADH. Thus conditions that affect the ability to produce concentrated urine (e.g., diabetes insipidus, osmotic diuresis) contribute to the development of hypernatremia. Because sodium is the major determinant of ECF osmolality, hypernatremia always causes hypertonicity. In turn, hypertonicity causes a shift of water out of the cells, which leads to cellular dehydration. Dehydration of cerebral cells results in the development of central nervous system (CNS) symptoms.

## Assessment

1. **Signs and symptoms:** Intense thirst, fatigue, restlessness, irritability, altered mental status, high pitched cry in the infant, and coma. Symptomatic hypernatremia occurs only in individuals who do not have access to water or have an altered thirst mechanism (e.g., infants, older adults, those who are comatose).
2. **Physical assessment:** Low-grade fever, flushed skin, peripheral and pulmonary edema (sodium gain), postural hypotension and tachycardia (water loss), increased muscle tone and deep tendon reflexes, and muscle twitching and spasticity. Depressed anterior fontanelle and sunken eyes in the infant with hypernatremic dehydration.
3. **Hemodynamic measurements:** Variable.
   - *Sodium excess:* Increased CVP and PAP.
   - *Water loss:* Decreased CVP and PAP. The volume effects of water loss are minimized because of movement of water out of the cells as the result of hypernatremia-induced hypertonicity.

NOTE: Symptoms are most likely to develop with a sudden increase in plasma sodium to greater than 160 mmol/L. After approximately 24 hours, brain cells adjust to ECF hypertonicity by increasing intracellular osmolality. The exact mechanism by which this occurs is unclear, but it is known that this increased osmolality helps maintain cellular hydration. Thus individuals with chronic hypernatremia may have few symptoms. This adaptive mechanism has great significance in the treatment of hypernatremia. If the plasma sodium is reduced too quickly via administration of water, there is a rapid movement of water into the cells as a result of increased intracellular osmolality. The net result may be dangerous cerebral edema (see pp. 24-25).

4. **History and risk factors:**
   - *Water loss*

Increased insensible and sensible fluid loss (e.g., diaphoresis, respiratory infection)

Diabetes insipidus (see Chapter 20)

Osmotic diuresis (e.g., hyperglycemia)

Osmotic diarrhea (e.g., lactulose)

- *Water deprivation*

  Inadequate provision of water to patients with an impaired ability to regulate water intake (e.g., in cases of coma, tube feedings, or mechanical ventilation).

- *Sodium gain*

  IV administration of hypertonic saline solution or sodium bicarbonate

  Primary aldosteronism

  Saltwater near-drowning

  Drugs (e.g., sodium polystyrene sulfonate [Kayexalate])

  Hypernatremic dehydration in the breastfed neonate from failure to adequately establish lactation.

## Diagnostic Tests

1. **Plasma sodium:** Is greater than 145 mmol/L.
2. **Plasma osmolality:** Increased because of elevated serum sodium.
3. **Urine sodium:** Decreased with renal water loss (e.g., diabetes insipidus); increased with sodium gain.
4. **Urine specific gravity and osmolality:** Increased because of the kidneys' attempt to retain water; decreased in diabetes insipidus.
5. **Dehydration test**: Water withheld for 16 to 18 hours. Serum and urine osmolality then checked 1 hour after administration of ADH. This test is used to identify the etiology of polyuric syndromes (e.g., central versus nephrogenic diabetes insipidus).

## Collaborative Management

1. **IV or oral water replacement:** To treat water loss. If sodium is more than 160 mmol/L, IV 5% dextrose in water ($D_5W$) or hypotonic saline solution is given to replace pure water deficit.
2. **Diuretics in combination with oral or IV water replacement:** To treat sodium gain.

3. **Desmopressin acetate (DDAVP):** To treat central diabetes insipidus.
4. **Removal of cause:** Discontinuing medications such as lithium or correcting electrolyte imbalances such as hypokalemia and hypercalcemia to correct nephrogenic diabetes insipidus. Thiazide diuretics combined with a low-sodium diet may be prescribed for nephrogenic diabetes insipidus. Treating fever or diarrhea to minimize abnormal fluid loss.

NOTE: Hypernatremia is corrected slowly, over approximately 2 days, to avoid too great a shift of water into the brain cells.

## Nursing Diagnoses and Interventions

**Ineffective protection** related to altered sensorium from primary hypernatremia or cerebral edema occurring with too-rapid correction of hypernatremia.

**Desired outcomes:** The patient verbalizes orientation to time, place, and person and does not exhibit evidence of injury as a result of altered sensorium or seizures.

1. Cerebral edema may occur if hypernatremia is corrected too rapidly. Monitor serial plasma sodium levels. Sodium should not decrease at a rate greater than 0.5 to 1 mmol/L/hour. Sodium should be normalized over 24 to 48 hours in the patient with chronic hypernatremia. Consult with the physician regarding rapid decreases.
2. Assess the patient for indicators of cerebral edema: lethargy, headache, nausea, vomiting, increased BP, widening pulse pressure, decreased pulse rate, and seizures.
3. Assess and document LOC, orientation, and neurologic status with each check of VS. Reorient the patient as necessary. Alert the physician to significant changes.
4. Inform the patient and significant others that altered sensorium is temporary and improves with treatment.
5. Keep the side rails up and the bed in its lowest position, with the wheels locked.
6. Use reality therapy such as clocks, calendars, and familiar objects; keep these items at the bedside within the patient's visual field.
7. If seizures are anticipated, pad the side rails and keep an appropriate-size airway at the bedside.
8. Provide comfort measures to decrease thirst.

9. Weigh breastfed infants between 72 and 96 hours after birth to identify lactation failure. Infants at greatest risk for lactation failure are those born to first-time mothers or mothers with poor support for lactation. The infant with breastfeeding hypernatremic dehydration presents with weight loss, lethargy, dry mucous membranes, sunken eyes, and a depressed anterior fontanelle.

See pp. 73 and 76-78 for deficient fluid volume (applicable to hypernatremia caused by water loss); see pp. 80-84 for excess fluid volume (applicable to hypernatremia caused by sodium gain).

## Patient-Family Teaching Guidelines

Give the patient and significant others verbal and written instructions for the following:

1. Medications: name, purpose, dosage, frequency, precautions, and potential side effects. Teach signs and symptoms of hypokalemia if the patient is taking diuretics and review foods that are high in potassium (see Box 8-1).
2. Signs and symptoms of hypovolemia, if hypernatremia is related to abnormal fluid loss.
3. The importance of ensuring that infants and older adults are given adequate water to replace normal and abnormal losses (e.g., during hot weather).

# Disorders of Potassium Balance

8

Potassium is the primary intracellular cation and thus plays a vital role in cell metabolism. A relatively small amount (approximately 2%) of potassium is located within the extracellular fluid (ECF) and is maintained within a narrow range. Approximately 98% of the body's potassium is located within the cells. The sodium-potassium adenosine triphosphatase (ATPase) pump located in the cell membrane is critical to maintaining the balance between intracellular and extracellular potassium. The pump actively transports sodium out of the cell and potassium into the cell. Adequate intracellular magnesium is necessary for normal function of the pump. Because the ratio of intracellular fluid (ICF) potassium to ECF potassium helps determine the resting membrane potential of nerve and muscle cells, an alteration in the plasma potassium level may adversely affect neuromuscular and cardiac function.

Distribution of potassium between ECF and ICF is affected by ECF pH, insulin levels, and $beta_2$-adrenergic activity/agents (e.g., epinephrine). Increased insulin levels and stimulation of $beta_2$-adrenergic receptors cause an intracellular shift of potassium. Acute changes in serum pH are accompanied by reciprocal changes in serum potassium concentration. In acidosis, for example, excess hydrogen ions move into the cells to be buffered. To maintain electric neutrality within the cell, another positive ion (e.g., potassium) must move out. In alkalosis the reverse occurs. Hydrogen ions shift out of the cell and potassium ions shift in.

The body gains potassium through foods (primarily meats, fruits, and vegetables) and medications. In addition, ECF gains potassium any time there is a breakdown of cells (tissue catabolism) or a movement of potassium out of the cells. However, an elevated serum potassium level usually does not occur unless there is a concomitant reduction in renal function. Potassium is lost from the body through the kidneys (80%), gastrointestinal (GI) tract (15%), and skin (5%). Potassium may be lost from ECF because of an intracellular shift or tissue anabolism.

The kidneys are the primary regulators of potassium balance. They regulate this by adjusting the amount of potassium excreted in the urine. As the serum potassium level rises after a potassium load, so does the level in the renal tubular cell. This creates a concentration gradient that favors the movement of potassium into the renal tubule with the loss of potassium in the urine. Aldosterone, secreted by the adrenal cortex in response to an increased plasma potassium level, also increases urinary excretion of potassium. Thus conditions that increase aldosterone levels (e.g., volume depletion or postsurgical stress) may cause excessive loss of potassium. The rate of urine flow affects potassium excretion so that conditions associated with increased urine production may increase potassium loss. The kidneys are unable to conserve potassium as avidly as sodium, and a significant amount of potassium still may be lost in the urine in the presence of potassium depletion. Normal serum potassium is 3.5 to 5 milliequivalents/liter (mmol/L).

## Hypokalemia

Hypokalemia, one of the most common electrolyte disturbances, occurs because of an increased loss of potassium from the body or a movement of potassium into the cells and is rarely the result of inadequate intake alone. Conditions that cause volume depletion (e.g., abnormal GI losses) stimulate the release of aldosterone, resulting in increased loss of potassium in the urine. Hypomagnesemia may contribute to the development of hypokalemia as a result of increased movement of potassium out of cells and increased urinary excretion. Changes in serum potassium levels reflect changes in ECF potassium, not necessarily changes in total body levels.

## Assessment

1. **Clinical manifestations:** Fatigue, muscle weakness, leg cramps, soft and flabby muscles, nausea, vomiting, ileus, constipation, paresthesias, enhanced digitalis effect, and decreased urine concentration (i.e., nephrogenic diabetes insipidus). Severe hypokalemia can cause dysrhythmias, hypoventilation and paralysis.

2. **Physical assessment:** Decreased bowel sounds caused by smooth muscle weakness, weak and irregular pulse, decreased reflexes, and decreased muscle tone.

NOTE: Patients often have no symptoms, particularly when hypokalemia is mild. However, patients with existing cardiac disease are at risk for cardiac dysrhythmias with even mild hypokalemia.

3. **History and risk factors:**
   - *Reduction in total body potassium*
     Increased urinary losses: Diuretics, magnesium deficiency, osmotic diuresis, hyperaldosteronism (e.g., congenital adrenal hyperplasia), renal tubular acidosis
     Increased GI losses, especially gastric losses (e.g., pyloric stenosis, nasogastric [NG] suction)
     Increased loss through diaphoresis

NOTE: Poor dietary intake may contribute to, but rarely causes, hypokalemia. Hypokalemia may develop in the patient who is maintained on parenteral fluids with inadequate replacement of potassium.

   - *Intracellular shift*
     Increased insulin (e.g., from total parenteral nutrition [TPN], treatment of diabetic ketoacidosis [DKA])
     Alkalosis, or after correction of acidosis (e.g., treatment of DKA)
     During periods of tissue repair after burns, trauma, or starvation; usually accompanied by inadequate intake or replacement of potassium
     Administration of beta-adrenergic agonists (e.g., epinephrine, terbutaline, albuterol) or increased beta-adrenergic activity (e.g., stress, coronary ischemia)

## Diagnostic Tests

1. **Serum potassium:** Values are less than 3.5 mmol/L.

2. **Urine potassium:** Levels greater than 20 mmol/L indicate renal loss of potassium. Levels less than 20 mmol/L indicate hypokalemia from a nonrenal cause.
3. **Transtubular $K^+$ concentration gradient (TTKG):** A value calculated by dividing the ratio of urine potassium to serum potassium by the ratio of urine osmolality to serum osmolality. TTKG is used to evaluate the cause of increased urinary potassium levels.
4. **Arterial blood gases (ABGs):** May show metabolic alkalosis (increased pH and bicarbonate ion [$HCO_3^-$]) because hypokalemia is often associated with this condition (e.g., NG suction, diuretic therapy, hyperaldosteronism). Hypokalemia also may be associated with metabolic acidosis (e.g., diarrhea, renal tubular acidosis).
5. **Electrocardiogram (ECG):** ST-segment depression, flattened T wave, presence of U wave, and ventricular dysrhythmias (Figure 8-1). NOTE: Hypokalemia potentiates the effects of digitalis. ECG may reveal signs of digitalis toxicity in spite of a normal serum digitalis level.

## Collaborative Management

1. **Treatment of the underlying cause**
2. **Increased consumption of potassium-rich foods**
3. **Replacement of potassium:** Either by mouth (PO; via increased dietary intake or medication) or intravenously (IV). The usual dose is 40 to 80 mmol/day in divided doses. IV potassium is necessary if hypokalemia is severe or if the patient is unable to take potassium orally. IV potassium should not be administered at rates exceeding 10 to 20 mmol/hour or in concentrations higher than 30 to 40 mmol/L unless hypokalemia is severe because this can result in life-threatening hyperkalemia. If potassium is administered via a peripheral line, the rate of administration may need to be reduced to prevent irritation of vessels. Patients receiving greater than 10 mmol/hour should be on a continuous cardiac monitor. The development of peaked T waves suggests the presence of hyperkalemia and requires immediate physician notification. Potassium is NEVER administered with IV push. Although as little as 20 mmol/day is usually sufficient to prevent hypokalemia, 40 to 100 mmol/day is generally necessary to treat it.

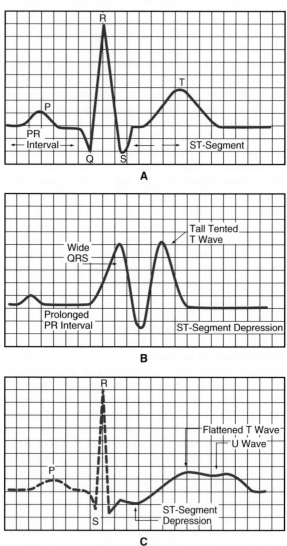

Figure 8-1
**A,** Normal ECG tracing. **B,** Serum potassium level above normal. **C,** Serum potassium level below normal.

Potassium is usually replaced in combination with chloride or phosphate. Because hypokalemia is frequently associated with ECF volume deficit and chloride loss (e.g., vomiting, diuretics), potassium chloride is usually the preparation of choice. When hypokalemia is associated with a need for intracellular anions (e.g., TPN or treatment of DKA), potassium phosphate may be the preferred preparation. In the treatment of DKA, when large volumes of isotonic sodium chloride (NaCl) are given, the phosphate preparation has the additional benefit of avoiding additional chloride administration. Hypokalemia associated with metabolic acidosis (e.g., renal tubular acidosis) may be treated with potassium bicarbonate or citrate.

4. **Potassium-sparing diuretics:** May be given in place of oral potassium supplements.
5. **Potassium chloride salt substitute:** May be used to supplement potassium intake (1 teaspoon equals approximately 60 mmol potassium chloride).
6. **Correction of magnesium depletion (if present):** Magnesium deficiency should be suspected when hypokalemia persists despite significant potassium replacement.

## Nursing Diagnoses and Interventions

**Decreased cardiac output** related to altered conduction (risk of ventricular dysrhythmias) from hypokalemia or too-rapid correction of hypokalemia with resulting hyperkalemia.

**Desired outcomes:** ECG shows normal configuration and absence of ventricular dysrhythmias. Pulse rate and rhythm are normal for the patient. Serum potassium levels are within the normal range (3.5 to 5 mmol/L).

1. Administer IV potassium supplement as prescribed. Avoid giving IV potassium chloride at a rate faster than recommended because this can lead to life-threatening hyperkalemia (see p. 113). Potassium supplementation for symptomatic hypokalemia is usually given in isotonic saline because 5% dextrose in water ($D_5W$) increases insulin-induced intracellular shift of potassium. Concentrated solutions of potassium may be hung in limited volumes (e.g., 20 mmol in 100 milliliters [mL] of NaCl), but it should be administered no more rapidly than 20 mmol/hour. Concentrated solutions and infusion rates

of greater than 10 mmol/hour are used only with severe hypokalemia. Do not add potassium chloride to IV solution containers in the hanging position because this can cause layering of the medication. Instead, invert the solution container before adding the medication and mix well.

IV potassium chloride can cause local irritation of veins and chemical phlebitis. Assess IV insertion site for erythema, heat, or pain. Consult with the physician if symptoms develop. Irritation may be relieved by applying an ice bag, giving mild sedation, or numbing the insertion site with a small amount of local anesthetic. Phlebitis may necessitate changing the IV site.

2. Administer oral potassium supplements as prescribed. NOTE: Oral supplements may cause GI irritation. Administer with a full glass of water or fruit juice; encourage the patient to sip slowly. Consult with the physician if symptoms of abdominal pain, distention, nausea, or vomiting develop. Do not switch potassium supplements without a physician's prescription.

3. Administer magnesium supplements as prescribed. NOTE: Combined potassium and magnesium deficiencies have been associated with increased frequency of dysrhythmias and mortality in cases of acute myocardial infarction (see Chapter 11).

4. Encourage intake of foods high in potassium (Box 8-1). Salt substitutes may be used as an inexpensive potassium supplement.

5. Monitor intake and output (I&O) hourly. Alert the physician to a urine output of less than 0.5 mL/kilogram [kg]/hour. Unless severe symptomatic hypokalemia is present, potassium supplements should not be given if the patient has an inadequate urine output because hyperkalemia can develop rapidly in patients with oliguria (< 15 to 20 mL/hour). Increased urine output increases the risk for hypokalemia.

6. Monitor for the presence of an irregular pulse or pulse deficit (a discrepancy between the apical and radial pulse rates). Alert the physician to changes. Individuals with a history of heart failure, myocardial ischemia, or previous dysrhythmias are at particular risk for hypokalemia-induced dysrhythmias.

## Box 8-1    Foods High in Potassium

- Apricots
- Artichokes
- Avocados
- Bananas
- Cantaloupe
- Carrots
- Chocolate
- Dried beans and peas
- Dried fruit
- Meat
- Melons
- Mushrooms
- Nuts
- Oranges, orange juice
- Potatoes
- Prune juice
- Pumpkin
- Rhubarb
- Salt substitute
- Spinach
- Sweet potatoes
- Swiss chard
- Tomatoes, tomato juice, tomato sauce
- Turnips

7. Physical indicators of abnormal potassium levels are difficult to identify in a patient who is critically ill. Monitor ECG for signs of continuing hypokalemia (ST-segment depression, flattened T wave, presence of U wave, ventricular dysrhythmias) or hyperkalemia (tall, thin T waves; prolonged PR interval; ST depression; widened QRS; loss of P wave), which may develop during potassium replacement (see Figure 8-1).

8. Monitor plasma potassium levels carefully, especially in individuals at risk for development of hypokalemia (e.g., patients taking diuretics or receiving NG suction). Monitor plasma magnesium levels in patients who do not respond to potassium replacement.

9. Administer potassium cautiously to patients receiving potassium-sparing diuretics (e.g., spironolactone amiloride, triamterene) or angiotensin-converting enzyme (ACE) inhibitors (e.g., captopril) because of the potential for the development of hyperkalemia.

10. Because hypokalemia can potentiate the effects of digitalis, monitor patients receiving digitalis for signs of increased digitalis effect: multifocal or bigeminal premature ventricular contractions (PVCs), paroxysmal atrial tachycardia with varying atrioventricular (AV) block, and other heart blocks.

11. Monitor patients for continued risk for hypokalemia (e.g., aggressive insulin administration, use of beta-adrenergic medications, increased urine output, diarrhea, vomiting,) or worsening symptoms.

**Ineffective breathing pattern** (or risk for) related to weakness or paralysis of respiratory muscles from severe hypokalemia (potassium < 2 to 2.5 mmol/L).

**Desired outcome:** The patient has an effective breathing pattern as evidenced by normal respiratory depth, pattern, and rate of 12 to 20 breaths/minute.

1. If the patient has signs of worsening hypokalemia, be aware that severe hypokalemia can lead to weakness of respiratory muscles, resulting in shallow respirations and, eventually, apnea and respiratory arrest. Assess character, rate, and depth of respirations. Alert the physician promptly if respirations become rapid and shallow.
2. Keep a manual resuscitator at the patient's bedside if severe hypokalemia is suspected.
3. Reposition the patient every 2 hours to prevent stasis of secretions; suction airway as needed.

## Patient-Family Teaching Guidelines

Give the patient and significant others verbal and written instructions for the following:

1. Medications: name, purpose, dosage, frequency, precautions, and potential side effects. Teach the patient the importance of taking prescribed potassium supplements if taking diuretics or digitalis. Review the indicators of digitalis toxicity.
2. Indicators of hypokalemia and hyperkalemia.
3. Foods that are high in potassium (see Box 8-1); use of salt substitute to supplement potassium, if appropriate.

## Hyperkalemia

Hyperkalemia (serum potassium level > 5 mmol/L) occurs because of an increased intake of potassium, a decreased urinary excretion of potassium, or movement of potassium out of the cells. Changes in serum potassium levels reflect changes in ECF potassium, not necessarily changes in total body levels. In DKA, for example, the patient initially may have elevated serum potassium despite the loss of a large quantity of potassium in the urine. This occurs because of the shift of potassium out of the cells as a result of a lack of insulin, increased tissue catabolism, and acidosis. (For additional information, see Chapter 20.) Chronic hyperkalemia is usually the result of decreased urinary excretion of potassium.

## Assessment

1. **Clinical manifestations:** Irritability, anxiety, abdominal cramping, diarrhea, weakness (especially of lower extremities), and paresthesias.
2. **Physical assessment:** Irregular pulse; cardiac standstill if hyperkalemia is sudden or severe.
3. **History and risk factors:**
   - *Inappropriately high intake of potassium:* Usually through IV potassium delivery
   - *Decreased excretion of potassium*
     Renal failure, acute and chronic (glomerular filtration rate [GFR] < 10% to 20% of normal)
     Use of potassium-sparing diuretics, ACE inhibitors, or nonsteroidal antiinflammatory drugs (NSAIDs)
     Adrenal insufficiency (Addison's disease)
     Syndrome of hyporeninemic hypoaldosteronism
   - *Movement of potassium out of the cells*
     Acidosis, both metabolic and respiratory
     Insulin deficiency, especially in patients with chronic renal failure
     Tissue catabolism (e.g., with fever, sepsis, trauma, or surgery)
     Hypertonic states (e.g., uncontrolled diabetes)

The severity of symptoms depends on the rate of change in the serum potassium level and the overall level.

## Diagnostic Tests

1. **Serum potassium:** Is more than 5 mmol/L. Several factors may cause a falsely high serum potassium because of increased release of intracellular potassium in the laboratory specimen (e.g., a high platelet count, prolonged use of a tourniquet and hand clinching at the time of venipuncture, hemolysis of the blood specimen, delayed separation of plasma and cells).

2. **TTKG:** A value calculated by dividing the ratio of urine potassium to serum potassium by the ratio of urine osmolality to serum osmolality. The TTKG is greater than 5 if the kidneys are capable of increasing excretion of potassium.
3. **Diagnostic ECG:** Progressive changes include tall, thin T waves; prolonged PR interval; ST depression; widened QRS; and loss of P wave. Eventually, QRS widens further (sine wave) and cardiac arrest occurs (see Figure 8-1).
4. **Serum cortisol or cortisone stimulation test:** Used for the diagnosis of Addison's disease.
5. **ABGs:** May show metabolic acidosis (decreased pH and $HCO_3^-$) because hyperkalemia often occurs with acidosis.

## Collaborative Management

The goal is to treat the underlying cause and return the serum potassium level to normal.

### Subacute

1. **Cation exchange resins (e.g., Kayexalate):** Given PO, NG, or via retention enema to exchange sodium for potassium in the bowel. The solution is usually combined with sorbitol to prevent constipation from the Kayexalate and induce diarrhea, thus increasing potassium loss in the bowels. Resins have a faster onset of action when given rectally. NOTE: Kayexalate may bind with other cations in the GI tract and contribute to the development of hypomagnesemia or hypocalcemia. Other complications of Kayexalate include sodium retention and fluid overload.
2. **Reduced potassium intake:** A diet avoiding foods high in potassium (see Box 8-1). Special enteral formulas low in potassium are available for patients with renal failure.
3. **Discontinuation of medications that increase the risk of hyperkalemia:** Salt substitutes, potassium supplements, potassium-sparing diuretics, ACE inhibitors, NSAIDs, heparin, beta-blocking agents.
4. **Fludrocortisone:** A mineralocorticoid that increases urinary excretion of potassium.

### Acute

1. **IV calcium gluconate:** To counteract the neuromuscular and cardiac effects of hyperkalemia. Serum potassium

levels remain elevated. Calcium chloride may also be used. NOTE: Calcium chloride and calcium gluconate are not interchangeable. Although both come in 10-mL ampules, calcium gluconate contains only 4.5 mEq of calcium, whereas calcium chloride contains 13.6 mEq of calcium. Effects of IV calcium should be evident within a few minutes of administration but last for only 30 to 60 minutes.

2. **IV glucose and insulin:** To shift potassium into the cells. This reduces serum potassium temporarily (for approximately 6 hours). Usually hypertonic glucose (either an amp of $D_{50}W$ or 250 to 500 mL of $D_{10}W$) is given with 10 to 15 units of regular insulin.

3. **Sodium bicarbonate ($NaHCO_3$):** To shift potassium into the cells. Reduces serum potassium temporarily (for approximately 1 to 2 hours).

4. **Beta$_2$ agonists:** To shift potassium into the cells. Albuterol or salbutamol may be administered through nasal inhalation or IV. IV administration should be used cautiously in patients with known coronary artery disease because of the risk of tachydysrhythmias and myocardial ischemia.

NOTE: The effects of calcium, glucose and insulin, beta$_2$ agonists, and $NaHCO_3$ are temporary. Usually it is necessary to follow these medications with a therapy that removes potassium from the body (e.g., dialysis, administration of cation exchange resins).

5. **Dialysis:** To remove potassium from the body. Dialysis is the most effective means of removing excess potassium.

## Nursing Diagnoses and Interventions

**Decreased cardiac output** (or risk for) related to altered conduction (risk of ventricular dysrhythmias) from severe hyperkalemia or too-rapid correction of hyperkalemia with resulting hypokalemia.

**Desired outcomes:** ECG shows no evidence of ventricular dysrhythmias related to hypokalemia (U wave, PVCs) or hyperkalemia (peaked T wave). Serum potassium levels are within the normal range (3.5 to 5 mmol/L).

1. Monitor I&O. Consult with the physician for a urine output less than 0.5 mL/kg/hour. Oliguria increases the risk for development of hyperkalemia.

2. Monitor for indicators for hyperkalemia (e.g., irritability, anxiety, abdominal cramping, diarrhea, weakness of lower extremities, paresthesias, irregular pulse). Also be alert to indicators of hypokalemia (e.g., fatigue, muscle weakness, leg cramps, nausea, vomiting, decreased bowel sounds, paresthesias, weak and irregular pulse) after treatment. Assess for hidden sources of potassium: medications (e.g., potassium penicillin G), banked blood (the older the blood, the greater the amount of potassium because of the release of potassium as red blood cells [RBCs] die and break down), salt substitute, GI bleeding, or conditions causing increased catabolism such as infection or trauma.

3. Monitor serum potassium levels, especially in patients at risk of development of hyperkalemia (e.g., individuals with renal failure). Consult with the physician for levels above or below the normal range. Monitor other laboratory values that may affect potassium levels (e.g., blood urea nitrogen [BUN], creatinine, ABG values, glucose).

4. Physical indicators of abnormal potassium levels are difficult to identify in a patient who is critically ill. Monitor ECG for signs of hypokalemia (ST-segment depression, flattened T waves, presence of U wave, ventricular dysrhythmias), which may develop from therapy, or continuing hyperkalemia (tall, thin T waves; prolonged PR interval; ST depression; widened QRS; loss of P wave). Consult a physician immediately if ECG changes occur. ECG changes at a given potassium level are less dramatic in the patient with chronic renal failure in whom hyperkalemia develops more slowly. (See Figure 8-1 for ECG changes associated with hypokalemia and hyperkalemia.)

5. Administer glucose and insulin in the order prescribed. When glucose is administered first, it stimulates endogenous insulin release and may potentiate the potassium-lowering effect of the exogenous insulin.

6. Administer calcium gluconate as prescribed, giving it cautiously to patients receiving digitalis because digitalis toxicity can occur. NOTE: Do not add calcium gluconate to solutions containing $NaHCO_3$ because precipitates may form. However, IV glucose and $NaHCO_3$ may be combined without harmful precipitates. Insulin should be given

separately. (For more information about calcium administration, see p. 127.)

7. If administering cation exchange resins by enema, encourage the patient to retain the solution for at least 30 to 60 minutes to ensure therapeutic effects. Administer Kayexalate (without sorbitol) via a Foley catheter inserted into the rectum. The balloon is filled with sterile water to keep the catheter in place, and the catheter is clamped. Cleansing enemas are recommended before administration to enhance absorption and afterward to reduce the risk of bowel complications. Follow specific institution policy.

## Patient-Family Teaching Guidelines

Give the patient and significant others verbal and written instructions for the following:

1. Medications: name, purpose, dosage, frequency, precautions, and potential side effects.

2. Indicators of both hypokalemia and hyperkalemia. Alert the patient to the following signs and symptoms that necessitate immediate medical attention: weakness and pulse irregularities. Teach the patient and significant others how to measure pulse rate and detect irregularities.

3. Foods high in potassium, which should be avoided (see Box 8-1). Remind the patient that salt substitute and "Lite" salt should also be avoided. Fruits that are relatively low in potassium include apples, grapes, and cranberries.

4. Importance of preventing recurrent hyperkalemia; review potential causes.

# Disorders of Calcium Balance

9

Calcium, one of the body's most abundant ions, primarily is combined with phosphorus to form the mineral salts of the bones and teeth. In addition, calcium exerts a sedative effect on nerve cells and has important intracellular functions, including development of the cardiac action potential and contraction of muscles. Less than 1% of the body's calcium is contained within extracellular fluid (ECF), yet this concentration is regulated carefully by parathyroid hormone, metabolites of vitamin D, and calcitonin. Parathyroid hormone is released by the parathyroid gland in response to a low-serum calcium level. It increases resorption of bone (movement of calcium and phosphorus out of the bone); activates vitamin D, which increases the absorption of calcium from the gastrointestinal (GI) tract; and stimulates the kidneys to conserve calcium and excrete phosphorus. Calcitonin is produced by the thyroid gland when serum calcium levels are elevated; it inhibits bone resorption.

The ECF gains calcium from intestinal absorption of dietary calcium and resorption of bones. It is lost from the ECF via secretion into the GI tract, urinary excretion, and deposition in the bone; a small amount is lost in sweat. Other than a transient increase during adolescence and pregnancy, the amount of calcium that is absorbed from the intestinal tract is limited to only about 20% to 30% of the calcium contained in foods and supplements. Inadequate calcium intake is associated with decreased bone density and osteoporosis, increased risk of colorectal cancer, and increased risk of hypertension. The serum calcium level cannot be used to evaluate the adequacy of dietary calcium intake because plasma levels are maintained even in the face of poor oral intake through the movement of calcium out of the bone.

Calcium is present in three different forms in the plasma: ionized, bound, and complexed. Approximately half of the plasma calcium is free ionized calcium. Slightly less than half the plasma calcium is bound to protein, primarily to albumin. The remaining small percentage is combined with nonprotein anions such as phosphate, citrate, and carbonate. Only the ionized calcium is physiologically important. Plasma pH, phosphorus, and albumin levels affect the percentage of calcium that is ionized. Therefore these factors must be considered in evaluation of total calcium levels.

The relationship between ionized calcium and plasma pH is reciprocal—an increase in pH decreases the percentage of calcium that is ionized. Patients with alkalosis (an increased pH), for example, may show signs of hypocalcemia despite a normal total calcium level (bound, complexed, and ionized). The relationship between plasma phosphorus and ionized calcium is also reciprocal. Changes in the plasma albumin level affect the total serum calcium level without changing the level of free calcium. In hypoalbuminemia, less protein is available to bind with calcium and the total calcium level drops; however, the level of ionized calcium is unchanged.

# Hypocalcemia

Symptomatic hypocalcemia may occur because of a reduction of total body calcium or of the percentage of calcium that is ionized. Total calcium levels may be decreased as a result of increased calcium loss, reduced intake from altered intestinal absorption, or altered regulation (e.g., hypoparathyroidism). Elevated phosphorus levels and decreased magnesium levels may precipitate hypocalcemia. Calcium and phosphorus have a reciprocal relationship: as one goes up, the other tends to go down. Hypomagnesemia may cause hypocalcemia as a result of the decreased action of the parathyroid hormone.

The most common cause of a low total calcium level is hypoalbuminemia. However, if the level of ionized calcium remains normal, the condition is asymptomatic and no treatment is necessary. In the presence of a decreased serum albumin level, treatment should be based on ionized calcium levels.

## Assessment

1. **Clinical manifestations:** Numbness with tingling of fingers and circumoral region, hyperactive reflexes, muscle cramps,

tetany, and convulsions. Lethargy and poor feeding may be present in the newborn. Alterations in mental status may include anxiety, depression, and frank psychosis. In chronic hypocalcemia, fractures may be present as a result of bone porosity. Sudden precipitous drops in plasma calcium levels may cause hypotension from vasodilation and heart failure from decreased myocardial contractility.

2. **Physical assessment**:
   - *Positive Trousseau's sign:* Ischemia-induced carpal spasm. It is elicited by applying a blood pressure (BP) cuff to the upper arm and inflating it past systolic BP for 2 minutes.
   - *Positive Chvostek's sign:* Unilateral contraction of facial and eyelid muscles. It is elicited by irritating the facial nerve by tapping the face just in front of the ear.

3. **Electrocardiogram (ECG) changes:** Prolonged QT interval caused by elongation of ST segment; may develop into a form of ventricular tachycardia called *torsades de pointes.*
   NOTE: The symptoms of hypocalcemia correlate with both the magnitude and rapidity of the fall in serum calcium. Thus a rapid drop in serum calcium is more likely to result in symptoms, at a given calcium level, than a gradual decline.

4. **History and risk factors:**
   - *Decreased ionized calcium*
     Alkalosis
     Administration of large quantities of citrated blood (citrate added to the blood to prevent clotting may bind with calcium, causing hypocalcemia)
     Hemodilution (e.g., caused by volume replacement with normal saline solution after hemorrhage)
     Hyperphosphatemia (e.g., renal failure, tumor lysis syndrome, rhabdomyolysis)
   - *Increased calcium loss in body fluids*
     Loop diuretics
   - *Decreased intestinal absorption*
     Decreased oral intake
     Impaired vitamin D metabolism (e.g., renal failure) or deficiency
     Chronic diarrhea
   - *Hypoparathyroidism*
     Congenital or acquired
   - *Hypomagnesemia*

- *Acute pancreatitis*
- *Chronic alcoholism*
- *Post partial parathyroidectomy or thyroidectomy for thyrotoxicosis*: Resulting from rapid movement of calcium back into the bone (hungry bone syndrome)

## Diagnostic Tests

1. **Total serum calcium level:** May be less than 8.5 milligrams/deciliter (mg/dL). If symptomatic hypocalcemia is the result of a reduction in the percentage of calcium that is ionized, the total serum calcium level is unchanged. Total serum calcium levels should be evaluated in relation to serum albumin and pH. For every 1 gram (g)/dL drop in the serum albumin level, there is a 0.8 to 1 mg/dL drop in total calcium level with no change in ionized calcium. For each 0.1 increase in pH, ionized calcium falls by approximately 0.2 mg/dL with no change in total calcium.
2. **Ionized serum calcium:** Is less than 4.5 mg/dL. Ionized calcium is the preferred test.
3. **Parathyroid hormone:** Decreased levels occur in hypoparathyroidism; increased levels may occur with other causes of hypocalcemia. Normal range is 150 to 350 picograms (pg)/mL (varies among laboratories).
4. **Magnesium and phosphorus levels:** May be checked to identify potential causes of hypocalcemia.

## Collaborative Management

1. **Treatment of the underlying cause**
2. **Calcium replacement:** Hypocalcemia is treated with oral (PO) or intravenous (IV) calcium. Patients with symptomatic hypocalcemia or corrected total calcium levels of less than 7.5 mg/dL usually need parenteral calcium. Tetany in adults is treated with 10 to 20 milliliters (mL) of 10% calcium gluconate IV or a continuous drip of 100 mL of 10% calcium gluconate in 1000 mL 5% dextrose in water ($D_5W$), infused over at least 4 hours.
3. **Magnesium replacement in individuals with magnesium deficiency:** Hypomagnesemia-induced hypocalcemia is often refractory to calcium therapy alone.
4. **Vitamin D and Vitamin D analogs**: To increase calcium absorption from the GI tract (Table 9-1). These preparations

Table 9-1   Vitamin D preparations and analogs

| Generic Name | Trade Name | Chemical Abbreviation |
| --- | --- | --- |
| Calcifediol | Calderol | $25(OH)D_3$ |
| Calcitriol | Rocaltrol | $1,25(OH)_2D_3$ |
| | Calcijex | |
| Cholecalciferol | Delta D | $D_3$ |
| | Vitamin $D_3$ | |
| Dihydrotachysterol | Hytakerol | DHT |
| Ergocalciferol | Calciferol | |
| | Vitamin D | |
| | Deltalin Gelseals | $D_2$ |

must be combined with adequate calcium intake to be effective.

5. **Aluminum hydroxide, calcium acetate, calcium carbonate antacids, or sevelamer hydrochloride**: To reduce an elevated phosphorus level before treatment of hypocalcemia in the patient with chronic renal failure (CRF).

6. **Increased dietary intake of calcium:** At least 1000 to 1500 mg/day for adults.

7. **Oral calcium supplements (e.g., calcium carbonate)**

## Nursing Diagnoses and Interventions

**Ineffective protection** (risk of tetany and seizures) related to neurosensory alterations from severe hypocalcemia.

**Desired outcomes:** The patient does not have evidence of injury caused by complications of severe hypocalcemia. Serum calcium levels are within normal range (total calcium: 8.5 to 10.5 mg/dL and ionized calcium 4.5 to 5.1 mg/dL).

1. Monitor the patient for evidence of worsening hypocalcemia: numbness and tingling of fingers and circumoral region, hyperactive reflexes, and muscle cramps. Consult with the physician promptly if these symptoms develop because they occur before overt tetany. In addition, consult with the physician if the patient has positive Trousseau's or Chvostek's signs because they also signal latent tetany. Monitor total and ionized calcium levels as available.

2. Administer IV calcium with caution. IV calcium should not be given faster than 0.5 to 1 mL/minute because rapid

## Box 9-1   Foods High in Calcium

- Brazil nuts
- Broccoli
- Cheese
- Collard, mustard, and turnip greens
- Cottage cheese
- Eggnog
- Ice cream
- Milk and cream
- Milk chocolate
- Molasses
- Oat flakes
- Rhubarb
- Seafood, especially canned sardines and canned salmon
- Sesame seeds
- Soy flour
- Spinach
- Tofu
- Yogurt

administration can cause hypotension. Observe the IV insertion site for evidence of infiltration because calcium sloughs tissue. Concentrated calcium solutions should be administered through a central line. Do not add calcium to solutions containing bicarbonate or phosphate because precipitates form. Digitalis toxicity may develop in patients taking digitalis because calcium potentiates its effects. Monitor the patient for signs and symptoms of hypercalcemia: lethargy, confusion, irritability, nausea, and vomiting. NOTE: Always clarify the type of IV calcium to be given. Both calcium chloride and calcium gluconate come in 10-mL ampules. One ampule of calcium chloride contains approximately 13.6 milliequivalents (mEq) of calcium, whereas an ampule of calcium gluconate contains 4.5 mEq of calcium.

3. For patients with chronic hypocalcemia, administer PO calcium supplements and vitamin D preparations (see Table 9-1) as prescribed. Because of the limited ability of the intestines to absorb calcium, supplements should be taken in multiple daily doses. Whether from food or supplements, the body cannot handle more than 500 mg at one time. Administer phosphorus-binding antacids with meals to ensure phosphorus binding.

4. Encourage intake of foods high in calcium: milk products, meats, and leafy green vegetables (Box 9-1).

5. Consult the physician if the response to calcium therapy is ineffective. Tetany that does not respond to IV calcium may be caused by hypomagnesemia.

6. Monitor for calcium loss (e.g., with loop diuretics, renal tubular dysfunction) or conditions that place the patient at risk (e.g., acute pancreatitis, acute alkalosis).
7. Keep symptomatic patients on seizure precautions; decrease environmental stimuli.
8. Avoid hyperventilation in patients in whom hypocalcemia is suspected. Respiratory alkalosis may precipitate tetany as a result of increased pH with a reduction in ionized calcium.
9. Inform the patient and significant others that the neuropsychiatric symptoms of hypocalcemia improve with treatment.

**Decreased cardiac output** related to altered conduction or decreased cardiac contractility from hypocalcemia or digitalis toxicity occurring with calcium replacement therapy.

**Desired outcomes:** The patient's cardiac output is adequate as evidenced by central venous pressure (CVP) 6 millimeters of mercury (mm Hg) or lower ($\leq 2$ centimeters of water [cm $H_2O$]), heart rate (HR) 100 beats per minute (bpm) or lower, BP within the patient's normal range, and absence of the clinical signs of heart failure or pulmonary edema (e.g., crackles, shortness of breath [SOB]). Critical care patients have a pulmonary artery pressure (PAP) of 20 to 30/8 to 15 mm Hg. ECG shows normal sinus rhythm without ectopy or other electrical disturbances.

1. Monitor ECG for signs of worsening hypocalcemia (prolonged QT interval) or digitalis toxicity with calcium replacement: multifocal or bigeminal premature ventricular contractions (PVCs), paroxysmal atrial tachycardia with varying atrioventricular (AV) block, and other heart blocks.
2. Hypocalcemia may decrease cardiac contractility. Monitor the patient for signs of heart failure or pulmonary edema: crackles (rales), rhonchi, SOB, decreased BP, increased HR, increased PAP, or increased CVP.

**Ineffective breathing pattern** related to laryngeal spasm occurring with severe hypocalcemia.

**Desired outcome:** The patient has respiratory depth, pattern, and rate (12 to 20 breaths/minute) within normal range and is asymptomatic of laryngeal spasm; symptoms of spasm include laryngeal stridor, dyspnea, or crowing.

1. Assess the patient's respiratory rate, character, and rhythm. Be alert to laryngeal stridor, dyspnea, and crowing, which

occur with laryngeal spasm, a life-threatening complication of hypocalcemia.
2. Keep an emergency tracheostomy tray at the bedside of symptomatic patients.

## Patient-Family Teaching Guidelines

Give the patient and significant others verbal and written instructions for the following:
1. Medications: name, purpose, dosage, frequency, precautions, and potential side effects.
2. Indicators of hypercalcemia and hypocalcemia. Review the symptoms that necessitate immediate medical attention: numbness and tingling of fingers and circumoral region and muscle cramps.
3. Foods that are high in calcium (see Table 9-1). Many foods that are high in calcium, such as milk products, also are high in phosphorus and may need to be limited in patients with renal failure. A program of phosphorus control and calcium supplementation may be necessary for patients who have renal failure.

# Hypercalcemia

Symptomatic hypercalcemia can occur because of an increase in total serum calcium or an increase in the percentage of free, ionized calcium. It typically develops with increased movement of calcium from the bone to the ECF (e.g., primary hyperparathyroidism and malignancy). If a normal or elevated serum phosphorus level accompanies hypercalcemia, calcium phosphate crystals may precipitate in the serum and deposit throughout the body. Soft tissue calcifications usually occur when the calcium-phosphorus product (i.e., serum calcium in mg/dL × serum phosphorus in mg/dL) exceeds 70.

## Assessment

1. **Clinical manifestations:** Symptoms are usually absent unless the calcium concentration is greater than 11 mg/dL. Symptoms include lethargy, weakness, anorexia, nausea, vomiting, polyuria (from nephrogenic diabetes insipidus), itching, bone pain, fractures, flank pain (from renal calculi),

depression, confusion, paresthesias, personality changes, stupor, and coma.

2. **ECG findings:** Shortening of ST segment and QT interval. PR interval is sometimes prolonged. Ventricular dysrhythmias can occur with severe hypercalcemia. There is an increased risk of digitalis toxicity.

3. **History and risk factors:**
   - *Increased release of calcium from bone*
     Hyperparathyroidism
     Malignant diseases from bone destruction or release of parathyroid hormone–like substances
     Prolonged immobilization
     Paget's disease
   - *Increased intestinal absorption*
     Vitamin D or A overdose
   - *Decreased urinary excretion*
     Renal failure
     Certain medications (e.g., thiazide diuretics)
   - *Increased intake of calcium*
     Excessive IV administration (e.g., for cardiopulmonary arrest)

## Diagnostic Tests

1. **Total serum calcium level:** May be greater than 10.5 mg/dL. The total calcium level should be evaluated with the serum albumin level. For a 1 g/dL drop in serum albumin level, there is a 0.8 to 1 mg/dL drop in total serum calcium.

2. **Ionized calcium:** Is more than 5.1 mg/dL.

3. **Parathyroid hormone:** Increased levels occur in primary or secondary hyperparathyroidism.

4. **Radiographic findings:** May reveal presence of osteoporosis, bone cavitation, or urinary calculi.

## Collaborative Management

NOTE: Mild, asymptomatic hypercalcemia often requires no treatment. Treatment of moderate hypercalcemia may depend on the severity of symptoms. Severe hypercalcemia (calcium level > 13.5 mg/dL) requires immediate treatment.

1. **Treatment of the underlying cause:** Antitumor chemotherapy for malignant disease or partial parathyroidectomy for hyperparathyroidism; discontinuation of calcium

supplements, vitamins A and D, and thiazide diuretics. In the patient with renal failure, vitamin D analogs such as doxercalciferol (Hectorol) or paricalcitol (Zemplar) used to treat and prevent secondary hyperparathyroidism need to be discontinued.

2. **IV normal saline solution:** Administered rapidly to increase urinary calcium excretion. Concomitant administration of furosemide prevents the development of fluid volume excess and further increases urinary calcium excretion.

3. **Low-calcium diet and cortisone:** To reduce intestinal absorption of calcium. Steroids compete with vitamin D, thereby reducing intestinal absorption of calcium. (For a list of foods high in calcium, see Box 9-1.)

4. **Pamidronate or etidronate:** Bisphosphates that inhibit bone resorption; used primarily to treat hypercalcemia associated with malignant disease. These medications are usually administered in 500 mL or more of saline solution over at least 4 hours to reduce the risk of nephrotoxicity. Bisphosphates take several days to work, but the effects may last for weeks.

5. **Plicamycin:** A cytotoxic antibiotic that acts directly on bone to reduce bone resorption. It is used primarily to treat hypercalcemia associated with neoplastic disease.

6. **Calcitonin:** To reduce bone resorption, increase bone deposition of calcium and phosphorus, and increase urinary calcium and phosphate excretion. Skin testing for allergy may be necessary before administration of salmon calcitonin.

7. **Gallium nitrate or zoledronic acid (Zometa):** Inhibit osteoclastic bone resorption; used in the treatment of malignant disease–induced hypercalcemia.

8. **Hemodialysis with a low calcium dialysate for the patient with renal failure**

9. **Partial parathyroidectomy for primary hyperparathyroidism**

## Nursing Diagnoses and Interventions

**Ineffective protection** related to neuromuscular changes resulting from hypercalcemia.

**Desired outcomes:** The patient does not have evidence of injury caused by neuromuscular or sensorium changes. The patient verbalizes orientation to person, place, and time. Serum calcium levels are within normal range (8.5 to 10.5 mg/dL; ionized calcium is 4.5 to 5.1 mg/dL).

1. Monitor the patient for worsening hypercalcemia. Assess and document the level of consciousness (LOC); patient's orientation to person, place, and time; and neurologic status with each vital sign (VS) check.

2. Personality changes, hallucinations, paranoia, and memory loss may occur with hypercalcemia. Inform the patient and significant others that altered sensorium is temporary and improves with treatment. Use reality therapy such as clocks, calendars, and familiar objects; keep them at the bedside within the patient's visual field.

3. Hypercalcemia causes neuromuscular depression with poor coordination, weakness, and altered gait. Provide a safe environment. Keep the side rails up and the bed in its lowest position, with the wheels locked. Assist the patient with ambulation if it is allowed.

4. Because hypercalcemia potentiates the effects of digitalis, monitor the patient taking digitalis for signs and symptoms of digitalis toxicity: anorexia, nausea, vomiting, and irregular pulse. ECG changes may include multifocal or bigeminal PVCs, paroxysmal atrial tachycardia with varying AV block, and other heart blocks. Monitor the patient for pulse changes in the non–ECG-monitored setting.

5. Monitor the serum electrolyte values for changes in serum calcium (normal range is 8.5 to 10.5 mg/dL); potassium (normal range is 3.5 to 5 mEq/L); and phosphorus (normal range is 2.5 to 4.5 mg/dL) as a result of therapy. Consult the physician regarding abnormal values. Correction of serum calcium levels may take several days to a week to achieve.

6. Administer saline and loop diuretics as prescribed. Evaluate the patient's response to therapy. Observe for signs of abnormal fluid volume.

7. Administer bisphosphates as prescribed. These medications are administered IV because of poor absorption from the GI tract. Monitor patients receiving pamidronate for fever, local reaction at infusion site, GI symptoms, and electrolyte imbalances (e.g., hypophosphatemia, hypokalemia,

hypomagnesemia). Consult with the physician regarding side effects.

8. Administer zoledronic acid IV over at least 15 minutes to reduce the risk of renal toxicity. Serum creatinine levels are recommended before and after medication administration.

9. Encourage increased mobility to reduce bone resorption. Ideally, the patient should be out of bed and up in a chair for at least 6 hours a day.

10. Avoid vitamin D preparations (see Table 9-1) because they increase intestinal absorption of calcium.

11. Provide the patient with a low-calcium diet and avoid the use of calcium-containing medications (e.g., antacids such as Tums).

**Impaired urinary elimination** related to dysuria, urgency, frequency, and polyuria from administration of diuretics, calcium stone formation, or changes in renal function occurring with hypercalcemia.

**Desired outcome:** The patient has a voiding pattern and urine characteristics that are normal for the patient.

1. Elevated urinary calcium levels may inhibit the kidneys' ability to concentrate urine (nephrogenic diabetes insipidus). This leads to polyuria and potential volume depletion. Monitor for signs of volume depletion, especially in patients receiving diuretics: decreased BP, CVP, and PAP and increased HR.

2. Monitor intake and output (I&O) hourly. Alert the physician to unusual changes in urine volume (e.g., oliguria alternating with polyuria), which may signal urinary tract obstruction, or continuous polyuria, which may be indicative of nephrogenic diabetes insipidus.

3. Because hypercalcemia can impair renal function, monitor the patient's renal function carefully: urine output, blood urea nitrogen (BUN), and creatinine.

4. Assess the patient for indicators of kidney stone formation: intermittent pain, nausea, vomiting, and hematuria. Encourage the intake of fruits (e.g., cranberries, prunes, plums) that leave an acid ash in the urine. An acidic urine reduces the risk of calcium stone formation. Also, increase fluid intake (at least 3 liters [L] in unrestricted patients) to reduce the risk of renal stone formation.

## Patient-Family Teaching Guidelines

Give the patient and significant others verbal and written instructions for the following:

1. Medications: name, purpose, dosage, frequency, precautions, and potential side effects.
2. Signs and symptoms of hypercalcemia.
3. Foods and over-the-counter medications (e.g., antacids) that are high in calcium. (See Box 9-1 for a list of foods high in calcium content.) Also, instruct patients to avoid vitamin supplements containing vitamins D and A.
4. If stone formation is a concern, the intake of foods that leave an acid ash in the urine. (Also, review the signs and symptoms of nephrolithiasis.)
5. After hospital discharge, the importance of increasing fluid intake (up to 4 L in nonrestricted patients) to minimize the risk of stone formation.
6. The importance of safe weight-bearing activities to decrease bone resorption.
7. For patients with malignant disease, the possible need for ongoing treatment of hypercalcemia.

# Disorders of Phosphorus Balance

10

Phosphorus is the primary anion of the intracellular fluid (ICF). Approximately 85% of the body's phosphorus is located in the bones and teeth, 14% is in the cells, and less than 1% is within the extracellular fluid (ECF). Because of the large intracellular store, in certain acute conditions, phosphorus may move into or out of the cell, causing dramatic changes in plasma phosphorus. Chronically, substantial increases or decreases can occur in intracellular phosphorus levels without significantly altering plasma levels. Thus plasma phosphorus levels do not necessarily reflect intracellular levels. Although most laboratories measure and report elemental phosphorus, nearly all the phosphorus in the body exists in the form of phosphate ($PO_4^{3-}$) and the terms *phosphorus* and *phosphate* often are used interchangeably.

Phosphorus is an important constituent of all body tissues and has a wide variety of vital functions, including formation of energy-storing substances (e.g., adenosine triphosphate [ATP]); formation of red blood cell (RBC) 2,3-diphosphoglycerate (DPG), which facilitates oxygen delivery to the tissues; metabolism of carbohydrates, protein, and fat; and maintenance of acid-base balance. In addition, phosphorus is critical to normal nerve and muscle function and provides structural support to bones and teeth. Plasma phosphorus levels vary with age, gender, and diet. Levels decrease with increasing age, with the exception of a slight rise in phosphorus in women after menopause. Glucose, insulin, or carbohydrate-containing foods cause a temporary drop in $PO_4^{3-}$ because of a shift of phosphorus into the cells.

Acid-base status also affects phosphorus balance. Alkalosis, particularly respiratory alkalosis, may cause hypophosphatemia as a result of an intracellular shift of phosphorus. The exact mechanism for this shift is not fully understood, but it may be related to an alkalosis-induced cellular glycolysis with increased formation of phosphorus-containing metabolic intermediates. Respiratory acidosis may cause a shift of phosphorus out of the cells and contribute to hyperphosphatemia.

Although the level of ECF phosphorus is regulated by a combination of factors, including dietary intake, intestinal absorption, and hormonally regulated bone resorption and deposition, balance depends largely on renal excretion. Parathyroid hormone (PTH) secretion results in increased absorption of phosphorus from the gastrointestinal (GI) tract and increased movement of phosphorus out of the bone. However, PTH also increases urinary excretion of phosphorus. Phosphorus balance is closely tied to that of calcium. The normal range for serum phosphorus is 2.5 to 4.5 milligrams/deciliter (mg/dL; 0.81 to 1.45 mmol/L).

## Hypophosphatemia

Hypophosphatemia (serum phosphorus < 2.5 mg/dL [0.81 mmol/L]) may be caused by transient intracellular shifts, increased urinary losses, decreased intestinal absorption, or increased cellular use (see the section on History and Risk Factors). Severe phosphorus deficiency may also occur with alcoholism, especially during acute withdrawal, from poor dietary intake, vomiting and diarrhea, hyperventilation, use of phosphorus-binding antacids, and increased urinary losses. In addition, a combination of factors may lead to hypophosphatemia in diabetic ketoacidosis (DKA). In DKA, a significant loss of phosphorus is seen in the urine because of the glucose-induced osmotic diuresis. This developing hypophosphatemia is masked, however, by the movement of phosphorus out of the cells as a result of increased tissue catabolism (cellular breakdown). When ketoacidosis is treated with glucose, insulin, and fluids, a dramatic shift of phosphorus back into the cells is seen and the existing phosphorus depletion then becomes apparent. (For more information about DKA, see Chapter 20.)

## Assessment

1. **Clinical manifestations:** Patients may be seen with acute symptoms caused by sudden decreases in serum phosphorus, or symptoms may develop gradually from chronic phosphorus deficiency. Most symptoms are the result of decreases in ATP and 2,3-DPG. Mild to moderate hypophosphatemia (1 to 2.5 mg/dL) is often asymptomatic; severe hypophosphatemia ($< 1$ mg/dL) may be potentially lethal because of altered cellular function.
   - *Acute:* Confusion, seizures, coma, chest pain from poor oxygenation of the myocardium, muscle pain, increased susceptibility to infection, numbness and tingling of the fingers and circumoral region, lack of coordination, and difficulty weaning from mechanical ventilation and respiratory failure.
   - *Chronic:* Memory loss, lethargy, and arthralgia.
2. **Physical assessment:**
   - *Acute:* Decreased strength as evidenced by difficulty speaking, weakness of respiratory muscles, and weakening hand grasp. Hypoxemia may cause an increased respiratory rate and respiratory alkalosis (from hyperventilation). Respiratory alkalosis causes phosphorus to move intracellularly, aggravating the existing hypophosphatemia. Bruising and bleeding may occur because of platelet dysfunction. Rhabdomyolysis, hemolysis, and myocardial depression may develop in severe hypophosphatemia.
   - *Chronic:* Weakness, joint stiffness, osteomalacia, cyanosis, and pseudofractures may occur.
3. **Hemodynamic measurements:** Patients with severe depletion may have signs of decreased myocardial function, including increased pulmonary artery wedge pressure (PAWP), decreased cardiac output (CO), and decreased blood pressure (BP), with decreased response to pressor agents.
4. **History and risk factors:**
   - *Intracellular shifts*
     Carbohydrate load
     Respiratory alkalosis (see Chapter 14)
     Total parenteral nutrition (TPN) with inadequate phosphorus content
     Androgen therapy

- *Increased use from increased tissue repair*
  Nutritional recovery, usually associated with TPN (see Chapter 26)
- *Increased urinary losses*
  Hypomagnesemia (see Chapter 11)
  Hypokalemia
  Hyperparathyroidism
  Use of thiazide diuretics
  Diuretic phase of acute tubular necrosis (ATN)
  Fanconi's syndrome
- *Reduced intestinal absorption or increased intestinal loss*
  Use of phosphorus-binding antacids (e.g., aluminum hydroxide, magnesium, or calcium-containing antacids)
  Vomiting, prolonged gastric suction, and diarrhea
  Malabsorption disorders, such as vitamin D deficiency
- *Mixed causes*
  Alcoholism and alcohol withdrawal
  DKA (with treatment)
  Severe burns

## Diagnostic Tests

1. **Serum phosphorus:** Less than 2.5 mg/dL (1.7 mEq/L)
   - *Moderate hypophosphatemia:* 1 to 2.5 mg/dL
   - *Severe hypophosphatemia:* Less than 1 mg/dL
2. **PTH level:** Elevated in hyperparathyroidism
3. **Serum magnesium:** May be decreased because of increased urinary excretion of magnesium in hypophosphatemia
4. **Alkaline phosphatase:** Increased with increased osteoblastic activity
5. **Radiographic films:** May reveal skeletal changes of osteomalacia or rickets

## Collaborative Management

1. **Identification and elimination of the cause:** For example, avoiding the use of phosphorus-binding antacids (e.g., aluminum, magnesium, or calcium antacids).
2. **Phosphorus supplementation:** Mild hypophosphatemia may be treated with increasing the intake of high-phosphorus foods, such as milk (Box 10-1). Mild to moderate hypophosphatemia usually can be treated with oral

---

### Box 10-1    Foods High in Phosphorus

- Meats, especially organ meats
  (e.g., brain, liver, kidney)
- Fish
- Poultry
- Milk and milk products
  (e.g., cheese, ice cream, cottage cheese)
- Whole grains (e.g., oatmeal, bran, barley)
- Seeds (e.g., pumpkin, sesame, sunflower)
- Nuts (e.g., Brazil nuts, peanuts)
- Eggs and egg products (e.g., eggnog, soufflés)
- Dried beans and peas

---

phosphate supplements such as Neutra Phos (sodium and potassium phosphate) or Phospho-Soda (sodium phosphate). Intravenous (IV) sodium phosphate or potassium phosphate is necessary in cases of severe hypophosphatemia or when the GI tract is nonfunctional.

## Nursing Diagnoses and Interventions

**Ineffective protection** related to sensory or neuromuscular dysfunction from hypophosphatemia-induced central nervous system (CNS) disturbances.

**Desired outcome:** The patient verbalizes orientation to person, place, and time and does not show evidence of injury caused by altered sensorium.

1. Monitor serum phosphorus levels in patients at increased risk; also monitor for associated electrolyte and acid-base imbalances: hypokalemia, hypomagnesemia, and respiratory alkalosis. Consult with the physician regarding abnormal levels.
2. Apprehension, confusion, and paresthesias are signals of developing hypophosphatemia. Assess and document the level of consciousness (LOC), orientation, and neurologic status with each vital sign (VS) check. Reorient the patient as necessary. Consult with the physician regarding significant changes.

3. Inform the patient and significant others that altered sensorium is temporary and improves with treatment.
4. Do not administer IV phosphate at a rate greater than that recommended by the manufacturer. Potential complications of IV phosphorus administration include tetany from hypocalcemia (serum calcium levels may drop suddenly if serum phosphorus levels increase suddenly [see pp. 124-125 for additional information]); soft tissue calcification (if the hyperphosphatemia develops, the calcium and phosphorus in the ECF may combine and form deposits in tissue [see p. 131]); and hypotension, caused by a too-rapid delivery. When IV phosphorus is administered as potassium phosphate, the infusion rate should not exceed 10 mEq/hour. Monitor the IV site for signs of infiltration because potassium phosphate can cause necrosis and sloughing of tissue (see pp. 113 and 115-116 for precautions when administering IV potassium).
5. Keep the side rails up and the bed in its lowest position, with the wheels locked.
6. Use reality therapy such as clocks, calendars, and familiar objects. Keep these articles at the bedside, within the patient's visual field.
7. If the patient is at risk for seizures, pad the side rails and keep an airway at the bedside.

**Impaired gas exchange** related to altered oxygen-carrying capacity of the blood from decreased 2,3-DPG and decreased gas exchange from decreased strength of respiratory muscles. NOTE: With decreased 2,3-DPG levels, the oxyhemoglobin dissociation curve shifts to the right. That is, at a given oxygen tension of arterial blood ($Pao_2$) level, more oxygen is bound to hemoglobin and less is available to the tissues.

**Desired outcome:** The patient exhibits normal respiratory function as evidenced by a resting rate of 12 to 20 breaths/minute with normal depth and pattern (eupnea) and an oxygen saturation of greater than 92%; normal skin color; absence of chest pain; and orientation to person, place, and time.

1. Monitor the rate and depth of respirations in patients who are severely hypophosphatemic. Consult with the physician regarding changes.

2. Assess the patient for signs of hypoxemia: restlessness, confusion, increased resting rate, symptoms of chest pain, and cyanosis (a late sign). Monitor arterial blood gas (ABG) values or oxygen saturation via pulse oximeter.

3. An increased incidence of hypophosphatemia is seen in patients with artificial ventilation. Monitor serum phosphate levels in these patients. Hypophosphatemia may contribute to difficulty in weaning patients from ventilators.

4. Administer phosphorus as prescribed.

**Impaired physical mobility** (or risk for) related to osteomalacia with bone pain and fractures caused by movement of phosphorus out of the bone from chronic hypophosphatemia or muscle weakness and acute rhabdomyolysis (breakdown of striated muscle) from severe hypophosphatemia.

**Desired outcome:** The patient has mobility without evidence of weakness, pain, or fractures.

1. Monitor all patients with suspected hypophosphatemia for evidence of decreasing muscle strength. Perform serial assessments of hand grasp strength and clarity of speech. Consult with the physician regarding changes.

2. Monitor serum phosphorus levels for evidence of worsening hypophosphatemia. Alert the physician to changes.

3. Assist the patient with ambulation and with activities of daily living. Keep personal items within easy reach.

4. Encourage the intake of foods high in phosphorus (see Box 10-1).

5. Medicate the patient for pain as prescribed.

**Decreased CO** related to negative inotropic changes associated with reduced myocardial functioning from severe phosphorus depletion.

**Desired outcomes:** The patient's CO is adequate as evidenced by central venous pressure (CVP) of less than 6 millimeters of mercury (mm Hg), heart rate (HR) of 100 or fewer beats per minute (bpm), BP within the patient's normal range, and absence of the clinical signs of heart failure or pulmonary edema. Critical care patients exhibit a pulmonary artery pressure (PAP) 20 to 30/8 to 15 mm Hg.

1. Monitor the patient for signs of heart failure or pulmonary edema: crackles (rales), rhonchi, shortness of breath (SOB), decreased BP, increased HR, increased PAP, or increased CVP.

2. Prevent the patient from hyperventilating if possible because respiratory alkalosis causes increased movement of phosphorus into the cells.

## Patient-Family Teaching Guidelines

Give the patient and significant others verbal and written instructions for the following:

1. Medications: name, purpose, dosage, frequency, precautions, and potential side effects.
2. Indicators of hypophosphatemia and hyperphosphatemia. Review the symptoms that necessitate immediate medical attention: weakness, SOB, and numbness and tingling of fingers and circumoral region. For patients at risk for chronic hypophosphatemia, warn of the need for notifying the physician of the presence of bone pain.
3. Foods that are high in phosphorus, if a high-phosphorus diet is encouraged (see Box 10-1).
4. The importance of using phosphorus-binding antacids only as prescribed by the physician.

# Hyperphosphatemia

Hyperphosphatemia (serum phosphorus >4.5 mg/dL [1.45 mmol/L]) occurs most often in the presence of renal insufficiency because of the kidneys' decreased ability to excrete excess phosphorus. In addition to renal failure, other causes of hyperphosphatemia include excessive intake of phosphates, extracellular shifts (i.e., movement of phosphorus out of the cell and into the ECF), cellular destruction with concomitant release of intracellular phosphorus, and decreased urinary losses that are unrelated to decreased renal function. As serum phosphorus levels increase, serum calcium levels often drop, which may cause hypocalcemia to develop (see Chapter 9). Hypocalcemia is most likely to occur in sudden, severe hyperphosphatemia (e.g., after IV administration of phosphates) or when the patient already is prone to hypocalcemia (e.g., with chronic renal failure).

The primary complication of hyperphosphatemia is metastatic calcification (i.e., the precipitation of calcium phosphate in the soft tissue, joints, and arteries). Precipitation of calcium phosphate occurs when the calcium-phosphorus product (calcium × phosphorus) exceeds 70. Chronic hyperphosphatemia in a patient with chronic renal failure may contribute to the development of renal osteodystrophy.

## Assessment

1. **Clinical manifestations:** Anorexia, nausea, vomiting, muscle weakness, hyperreflexia, tetany, and tachycardia. NOTE: Usually, patients have few symptoms with hyperphosphatemia. Most symptoms that do occur relate to the development of hypocalcemia or soft tissue (metastatic) calcifications. Indicators of metastatic calcification include oliguria, corneal haziness, conjunctivitis, irregular HR, and papular eruptions.

2. **Physical assessment:** See the section on Hypocalcemia, p. 125. In addition, see the previous Clinical Manifestations for indicators of metastatic calcifications.

3. **Electrocardiogram (ECG) changes:** See Hypocalcemia, p. 125. Deposition of calcium phosphate in the heart may lead to dysrhythmias and conduction disturbances.

4. **History and risk factors:**
   - *Decreased urinary excretion*
     Acute and chronic renal failure
     Hypoparathyroidism
     Volume depletion
   - *Increased intake*
     Excessive administration of phosphorus supplements
     Vitamin D excess with increased GI absorption
     Excessive use of phosphorus-containing laxatives or enemas (especially in children)
   - *Extracellular shift*
     Respiratory acidosis and metabolic acidosis
   - *Release from intracellular space*
     Neoplastic disease (e.g., leukemia, lymphoma), tumor lysis syndrome, and chemotherapy
     Increased tissue catabolism (breakdown)
     Rhabdomyolysis (breakdown of striated muscle) and crush injury

## Diagnostic Tests

1. **Serum phosphorus:** Is greater than 4.5 mg/dL (2.6 mEq/L) NOTE: Improper handling of blood specimens may result in

factitious (false) hyperphosphatemia because of hemolysis of blood cells.

2. **Serum calcium level:** Useful in assessment of potential consequences of treatment and diagnosis of primary problem
3. **Radiographic films:** May show skeletal changes of osteodystrophy
4. **Parathyroid hormone:** Level decreased in hypoparathyroidism
5. **Blood urea nitrogen (BUN) and creatinine:** For assessment of renal function

## Collaborative Management

1. **Identification and elimination of the cause:** For example, correction of volume depletion.
2. **Use of aluminum, magnesium, or calcium gels or antacids:** To bind phosphorus in the gut, thus increasing GI elimination of phosphorus (Table 10-1). NOTE: Magnesium antacids are avoided in renal failure because of the risk of hypermagnesemia. Calcium preparations are preferred in chronic renal failure because chronic use of aluminum preparations may contribute to the development of aplastic bone disease and aluminum dementia. Serum phosphorus levels may be allowed to remain slightly elevated (4.5 to

Table 10-1    Phosphorus-binding agents

| Agent | Trade Name | Dosage Form |
| --- | --- | --- |
| Aluminum carbonate | Basajel | Capsule |
| Aluminum hydroxide | Alternagel | Liquid |
| | Alucap | Capsule |
| | Amphojel | Liquid |
| | Dialume | Capsule |
| | Nephrox | Liquid |
| Calcium acetate | PhosLo | Tablet |
| | Phos-Ex | Tablet |
| Calcium carbonate | Caltrate | Tablet |
| | Os-Cal | Tablet |
| | Titralac | Liquid |
| | Tums | Tablet |
| Sevelamer hydrochloride | Renagel | Capsule |

6 mg/dL) in chronic renal failure to ensure adequate levels of 2,3-DPG. This helps limit the effects of chronic anemia on oxygen delivery to the tissues.

3. **Sevelamer hydrochloride (Renagel) capsules with meals:** To bind phosphorus in the gut; indicated for use in patients undergoing hemodialysis.

4. **Diet low in phosphorus:** See Box 10-1 for a list of foods that should be avoided or limited.

5. **Treatment of secondary hyperparathyroidism in chronic renal failure:** Excessive PTH production in chronic renal failure contributes to hyperphosphatemia and bone disease. Vitamin D preparations to reduce PTH levels: Paricalcitol (Zemplar), doxercalciferol (Hectorol) or calcitriol—oral (Rocaltrol) or IV (Calcijex). Paricalcitol and doxercalciferol have the advantage of not increasing intestinal absorption of calcium and phosphorus, thus allowing more aggressive treatment of hyperphosphatemia with calcium-binding antacids.

6. **Dialytic therapy:** May be necessary for acute, severe hyperphosphatemia accompanied by symptomatic hypo-calcemia.

## Nursing Diagnoses and Interventions

**Deficient knowledge** related to the purpose of phosphate binders and the importance of reducing GI absorption of phosphorus to control hyperphosphatemia and prevent long-term complications.

**Desired outcome:** The patient describes the potential complications of uncontrolled hyperphosphatemia and the ways in which they can be prevented. Because symptoms of hyperphosphatemia may be minimal, the prevention of long-term complications relies primarily on adequate patient education.

1. Teach patient the purpose of phosphate binders. Stress the need to take binders as prescribed with or after meals to maximize effectiveness. Calcium binders should be taken with the meal.

2. Prepare patient for the possibility of constipation from aluminum-binder use. Encourage the use of bulk-building supplements or stool softener if constipation occurs. Phosphate-containing laxatives and enemas must be avoided.

3. Phosphate binders are available in liquid or capsule form. Confer with the physician regarding an alternate form or brand for individuals who find binders unpalatable or difficult to take. Phosphate binders vary in their aluminum, magnesium, or calcium content, however, and one may not be exchanged for another without first ensuring that the patient is receiving the same amount of elemental aluminum, magnesium, or calcium.

4. Encourage the patient to avoid or limit foods high in phosphorus (see Box 10-1).

**Ineffective protection** related to precipitation of calcium phosphate in the soft tissue (e.g., cornea, lungs, kidneys, gastric mucosa, heart, blood vessels) and periarticular region of the large joints (e.g., hips, shoulders, elbows) or development of hypocalcemic tetany.

**Desired outcomes:** The patient exhibits no evidence of metastatic calcification or hypocalcemia. The calcium-phosphorus product (calcium × phosphorus) remains less than 70.

1. Monitor serum phosphorus and calcium levels. Consult with the physician regarding abnormal values. Remember that phosphorus values may be kept slightly higher (4.5 to 6 mg/dL) in patients with chronic renal failure to ensure adequate levels of 2,3-DPG, thereby minimizing effects of chronic anemia on oxygen delivery to the tissues.

2. Avoid vitamin D products (see Table 9-1) and calcium supplements until the serum phosphorus level approaches normal.

3. Alert the physician to indicators of metastatic calcification: oliguria, corneal haziness, conjunctivitis, irregular HR, and papular eruptions.

4. Monitor the patient for evidence of increasing hypocalcemia: numbness and tingling of the fingers and circumoral region, hyperactive reflexes, and muscle cramps. Notify the physician promptly if these symptoms develop because they may precede overt tetany. In addition, alert the physician if the patient has positive Trousseau's or Chvostek's signs because they signal latent tetany. (See p. 126 for a discussion of these signs and Chapter 9 for additional information regarding treatment and prevention of hypocalcemia.)

5. Because hyperphosphatemia can impair renal function, monitor the patient's renal function carefully: urine output,

BUN, and creatinine. (For additional information, see Chapter 22.)

## Patient-Family Teaching Guidelines

Give the patient and significant others verbal and written instructions for the following:

1. Medications: name, purpose, dosage, frequency, precautions, and potential side effects.
2. Indicators of hyperphosphatemia and hypocalcemia. Review the symptoms that require immediate medical attention: weakness, SOB, and numbness and tingling of fingers and circumoral region. Alert patients with chronic hyperphosphatemia to the necessity of notifying the physician if symptoms of metastatic calcification occur.
3. Foods that are high in phosphorus and thus must be avoided or limited (see Box 10-1).
4. The importance of avoiding phosphorus-containing over-the-counter medications: certain laxatives, enemas, and multivitamin and mineral supplements. Instruct the patient and significant others to read labels for the words *phosphorus* and *phosphate*.

# Disorders of Magnesium Balance

11

Magnesium is the body's fourth most abundant cation, yet its measurement and evaluation are often overlooked. Of the body's magnesium, approximately 50% to 60% is located in bone and approximately 1% is located in the extracellular fluid (ECF). The remaining magnesium is contained within the cells, constituting the second most abundant intracellular cation after potassium. Magnesium is regulated by a combination of factors, including vitamin D–controlled gastrointestinal (GI) absorption and renal excretion. Normally, only about 30% to 40% of dietary magnesium is absorbed. Renal excretion of magnesium changes to maintain magnesium balance and is affected by sodium and calcium excretion, ECF volume, and the presence of parathyroid hormone (PTH). Excretion of magnesium is decreased with increased PTH, decreased excretion of sodium or calcium, and fluid volume deficit.

Because magnesium is a major intracellular ion, it plays a vital role in normal cellular function. Specifically, it activates enzymes involved in the metabolism of carbohydrates and protein and triggers the sodium-potassium pump, thus affecting intracellular potassium levels. Magnesium is also important in the transmission of neuromuscular activity, neural transmission within the central nervous system (CNS), and myocardial functioning. Low magnesium intake has been identified as a risk factor for hypertension, cardiac dysrhythmias, ischemic heart disease, and sudden death. Low magnesium levels may contribute to the pathogenesis of coronary artery disease.

Approximately one fourth to one third of the plasma magnesium is bound to protein, a small portion is combined with other substances (complexed), and the remaining portion is free or ionized. It is the free ionized magnesium that is physiologically important. As with calcium levels, magnesium levels should be evaluated in combination with serum albumin levels. Low serum albumin levels decrease the total magnesium level, whereas the amount of free ionized magnesium may be unchanged. Magnesium may be used as a therapeutic agent in the treatment of preeclampsia-eclampsia, ischemic heart disease, dysrhythmias, or asthma. The normal range for serum magnesium is 1.5 to 2.5 milliequivalents/liter (mEq/L).

# Hypomagnesemia

Hypomagnesemia (serum magnesium level < 1.5 mEq/L) usually occurs because of a shift to the intracellular space, decreased GI absorption, or increased urinary loss. It also may occur with excessive GI loss (e.g., vomiting, diarrhea) or prolonged administration of magnesium-free parenteral fluids. Alcoholics (see the subsequent History and Risk Factors) and critical care patients are the two most common patient populations. In the critical care setting, hypomagnesemia is associated with increased mortality rates. Dysrhythmias and sudden death increase when decreased magnesium levels occur in combination with myocardial infarction, congestive heart failure, or digitalis toxicity. Hypomagnesemia is often associated with hypokalemia and hypocalcemia (see pp. 111 and 125, respectively, for additional information). Symptoms of hypomagnesemia tend to develop once the serum magnesium level drops to less than 1 mEq/L.

## Assessment

1. **Clinical manifestations:** Lethargy, weakness, fatigue, insomnia, mood changes, hallucinations, confusion, anorexia, nausea, vomiting, and paresthesias.
2. **Physical assessment:** Increased reflexes, tremors, convulsions, tetany, and positive Chvostek's and Trousseau's signs (see p. 126) in part caused by accompanying hypocalcemia. The patient also may have tachycardia, hypertension, and coronary spasm.
3. **Hemodynamic measurements:** See Hypokalemia, p. 111, and Hypocalcemia, p. 125.

4. **History and risk factors:**
   - *Chronic alcoholism:* Result of a combination of poor dietary intake, decreased GI absorption, and increased urinary excretion from ethanol effect
   - *Malabsorption syndrome*
     Cancer
     Colitis
     Pancreatic insufficiency
     Surgical resection of the GI tract
   - *Increased GI loss*
     Prolonged vomiting or gastric suction
     Prolonged diarrhea
   - *Administration of low-magnesium or magnesium-free parenteral solutions*
   - *Diabetic ketoacidosis (DKA) or poorly controlled diabetes:* Result of movement of magnesium out of the cell and loss in the urine because of osmotic diuresis from glucosuria
   - *Drugs that enhance urinary excretion*
     Loop diuretics
     Amphotericin
     Gentamicin
     Cisplatin
     Digoxin
     Cyclosporine
     Pentamidine
   - *Protein-calorie malnutrition*
   - *Intracellular shift*
     Insulin
     Catecholamine
     Hungry bone syndrome

## Diagnostic Tests

1. **Serum total magnesium level:** Is less than 1.5 mEq/L. Unfortunately, a normal serum total magnesium level does not eliminate the possibility of an intracellular deficiency.
2. **Serum ionized magnesium level:** A new test that provides a better indicator of intracellular magnesium because intracellular and extracellular levels of ionized magnesium are similar.

3. **Urinary magnesium level:** Helps identify renal causes of magnesium depletion; may be performed after parenteral administration of magnesium sulfate ($MgSO_4$; magnesium loading test).

4. **Serum albumin level:** A decreased albumin level may cause a decreased magnesium level because of a reduction in protein-bound magnesium. The amount of free ionized magnesium may be unchanged.

5. **Serum potassium level:** May be decreased because of failure of the cellular sodium-potassium pump to move potassium into the cell and the accompanying loss of potassium in the urine. This hypokalemia may be resistant to potassium replacement until the magnesium deficit has been corrected.

6. **Serum calcium level:** Hypomagnesemia may lead to hypocalcemia caused by a reduction in the release and action of PTH. PTH is the primary regulator of serum calcium levels (see Chapter 9).

7. **Electrocardiogram (ECG) evaluations:** May reflect magnesium, calcium, and potassium deficiencies, indicated by tachydysrhythmias, prolonged PR and QT intervals, widening of the QRS, ST-segment depression, and flattened T waves. Increased digitalis effect, as evidenced by multifocal or bigeminal premature ventricular contractions (PVCs), paroxysmal atrial tachycardia with varying atrioventricular (AV) block, and other heart blocks, also may occur. Dysrhythmias associated with hypomagnesemia include ventricular ectopy, torsades de pointes, and atrial fibrillation.

## Collaborative Management

1. **Identification and elimination of the cause:** For example, adequate replacement of magnesium in total parenteral nutrition (TPN) solutions.

2. **Intravenous (IV) or intramuscular (IM) $MgSO_4$:** For severe or symptomatic hypomagnesemia.

3. **Oral magnesium:** Magnesium oxide (Mag-Ox) or magnesium chloride (Slow-Mag) preparations may be used to treat mild or chronic hypomagnesemia. The dose is based on the amount of elemental magnesium contained in each preparation. Magnesium-containing antacids may also be used.

4. **Increased dietary intake of magnesium (Box 11-1).**

---

### Box 11-1    Foods High in Magnesium

- Green, leafy vegetables
  (e.g., beet greens, collard greens)
- Seafood and meat
- Nuts and seeds
- Wheat bran
- Soy flour
- Legumes
- Bananas
- Oranges
- Grapefruit
- Chocolate
- Molasses
- Coconuts

---

## Nursing Diagnoses and Interventions

**Ineffective protection** related to sensory or neuromuscular dysfunction as a result of hypomagnesemia.

**Desired outcomes:** The patient does not exhibit evidence of injury caused by complications of severe hypomagnesemia. Serum magnesium levels are within normal the range (1.5 to 2.5 mEq/L).

1. Monitor serum magnesium levels in patients at risk for development of hypomagnesemia (e.g., those who are alcohol abusers or who are receiving medications that increase urinary excretion). Consult with the physician regarding abnormal values. NOTE: Symptomatic hypomagnesemia may be mistakenly attributed to delirium tremens of chronic alcoholism. Be especially alert to indicators of magnesium deficit in these patients.

2. Administer IV $MgSO_4$ with caution. Refer to the manufacturer's guidelines. Too-rapid administration may lead to dangerous hypermagnesemia with cardiac or respiratory arrest. Patients receiving IV magnesium should be monitored for decreasing blood pressure (BP), labored respirations, and diminished patellar (knee jerk) reflex. An absent patellar reflex is a signal of hyporeflexia caused by dangerous hypermagnesemia. Should any of these changes occur, stop

the infusion and consult with the physician immediately (see pp. 158-159). Keep calcium gluconate at the bedside in the event of hypocalcemic tetany or sudden hypermagnesemia.

3. For patients with chronic hypomagnesemia, administer oral (PO) magnesium supplements as prescribed. All magnesium supplements should be given with caution in patients with reduced renal function because of an increased risk of the development of hypermagnesemia. Diarrhea is a common side effect of PO magnesium supplements. Consult with the physician if diarrhea develops.

4. Encourage the intake of foods high in magnesium in appropriate patients (see Box 11-1). NOTE: For most patients, a regular diet usually is adequate.

5. Keep symptomatic patients on seizure precautions. Decrease environmental stimuli (e.g., keep the room quiet, use subdued lighting).

6. Caution patients in whom hypocalcemia is suspected against hyperventilation. Respiratory alkalosis may precipitate tetany because of increased calcium binding.

7. Dysphagia may occur with hypomagnesemia. Test the patient's ability to swallow water before giving food or medications.

8. Assess and document the level of consciousness (LOC), orientation, and neurologic status with each vital sign (VS) check. Reorient the patient as necessary. Consult the physician regarding significant changes. Inform the patient and significant others that altered mood and sensorium are temporary and improve with treatment.

9. Consult with the physician for patients who are receiving magnesium-free solutions (e.g., TPN) for prolonged periods.

10. See Hypokalemia, pp. 111-118, and Hypocalcemia, pp. 125-131, for nursing care of these disorders. NOTE: Because magnesium is necessary for the movement of potassium into the cell, intracellular potassium deficits cannot be corrected until hypomagnesemia has been treated.

**Decreased cardiac output (CO)** related to electrical alterations associated with tachydysrhythmias or digitalis toxicity from hypomagnesemia.

**Desired outcome:** ECG shows normal configuration and the heart rate (HR) is within normal range for the patient. CO is adequate as evidenced by a CO greater than 4 L/minute. Patient exhibits brisk capillary refill and urinary output greater than 0.5 milliliters (mL)/kilogram (kg)/hour.

1. Monitor HR and regularity with each VS check. Consult the physician regarding changes. Be alert to decreased CO.
2. Assess the ECG in the patient on continuous ECG monitoring. Consider hypomagnesemia in patients in whom sudden ventricular dysrhythmias develop.
3. Because hypomagnesemia (and hypokalemia) potentiates the cardiac effects of digitalis, monitor patients taking digitalis for digitalis-induced dysrhythmias. ECG changes may include multifocal or bigeminal PVCs, paroxysmal atrial tachycardia with varying AV block, and other heart blocks. Monitor for pulse changes in the non-ECG monitored setting.
4. Monitor for and report decreased urinary output and delayed capillary refill.

**Imbalanced nutrition: less than body requirements** of magnesium related to history of poor intake or anorexia, nausea, and vomiting from hypomagnesemia.

**Desired outcome:** The patient verbalizes knowledge of foods high in magnesium content and shows consumption of these foods during meals.

1. Encourage the intake of small, frequent meals.
2. Teach the patient about foods high in magnesium content (see Box 11-1) and encourage the intake of these foods.
3. Medicate with antiemetics as prescribed.
4. Include the patient, significant others, and dietitian in meal planning as appropriate.
5. Provide oral hygiene before meals to enhance appetite.

## Patient-Family Teaching Guidelines

Give the patient and significant others verbal and written instructions for the following:

1. Medications: name, purpose, dosage, frequency, precautions, and potential side effects.
2. Indicators of hypomagnesemia, hypermagnesemia, and hypocalcemia. Emphasize the symptoms that necessitate immediate medical attention: numbness and tingling of

fingers and circumoral region, muscle cramps, altered sensorium, and irregular or rapid pulse.
3. Foods that are high in magnesium (see Box 11-1). Review the prescribed diet with the patient.
4. Referrals to Alcoholics Anonymous, Al-Anon, and Al-A-Teen as appropriate for an alcoholic patient and significant others.

# Hypermagnesemia

Hypermagnesemia (serum magnesium level $>2.5$ mEq/L) occurs almost exclusively in individuals with renal failure who have an increased intake of magnesium (e.g., use of magnesium-containing medications). It also may occur in acute adrenocortical insufficiency (Addison's disease) or during hypothermia. In rare cases, hypermagnesemia occurs because of excessive use of magnesium-containing medications (e.g., antacids, laxatives, enemas). The primary symptoms of hypermagnesemia are the result of depressed peripheral and central neuromuscular transmission. Symptoms usually do not occur until the magnesium level exceeds 4 mEq/L.

## Assessment

1. **Clinical manifestations:** Nausea, vomiting, flushing, diaphoresis, sensation of heat, altered mental functioning, drowsiness, coma, and muscular weakness or paralysis. Paralysis of the respiratory muscles may occur when the magnesium level exceeds 10 mEq/L.
2. **Physical assessment:** Hypotension, soft tissue (metastatic) calcification (see pp. 144-145), bradycardia, and decreased deep tendon reflexes. The patellar (knee jerk) reflex is lost once the magnesium level exceeds 8 mEq/L.
3. **Hemodynamic measurements:** Decreased arterial pressure because of peripheral vasodilation.
4. **History and risk factors:**
   ■ *Decreased excretion of magnesium*
   Renal failure
   Adrenocortical insufficiency
   ■ *Increased intake of magnesium*
   Excessive use of magnesium-containing antacids, enemas, and laxatives

Excessive administration of $MgSO_4$ (e.g., in the treatment of hypomagnesemia or preeclampsia-eclampsia)

## Diagnostic Tests

1. **Serum magnesium level:** Exceeds 2.5 mEq/L.
2. **ECG findings:** Prolonged QT interval and AV block may occur in severe hypermagnesemia (levels $> 12$ mEq/L).

## Collaborative Management

1. **Removal of cause:** For example, discontinuing or avoiding use of magnesium-containing medications or supplements, especially in patients with decreased renal function. (See Box 11-2 for a list of medications that contain magnesium.)
2. **Diuretics and 0.45% sodium chloride solution:** To enhance magnesium excretion in patients with adequate renal function.

---

### Box 11-2   Magnesium-Containing Medications

Antacids
Aludrox
Camalox
Di-Gel
Gaviscon
Gelusil and Gelusil II
Maalox and Maalox Plus
Mylanta and Mylanta II
Riopan
Simeco
Tempo

Magnesium-Containing Mineral Supplements
Laxatives

Magnesium citrate
Magnesium hydroxide
(milk of magnesium, Haley's M-O)
Magnesium sulfate (Epsom salts)

3. **IV calcium gluconate (10 mL of a 10% solution):** To antagonize the neuromuscular effects of magnesium for patients with potentially lethal hypermagnesemia.
4. **Dialysis with magnesium-free dialysate:** For patients with severely decreased renal function.

## Nursing Diagnoses and Interventions

**Ineffective protection** related to altered mental functioning, drowsiness and weakness, or metastatic calcification from hypermagnesemia.

**Desired outcomes:** The patient verbalizes orientation to person, place, and time and does not exhibit evidence of injury caused by complications of hypermagnesemia. The patient is asymptomatic of soft tissue (metastatic) calcifications: oliguria, corneal haziness conjunctivitis, irregular HR, and papular eruptions. Serum magnesium levels are within normal range (1.5 to 2.5 mEq/L).

1. Monitor serum magnesium levels in patients at risk for development of hypermagnesemia (e.g., those with chronic renal failure or women undergoing treatment for preeclampsia-eclampsia).
2. Assess and document LOC, orientation, and neurologic status (e.g., hand grasp) with each VS check. Assess patellar (knee jerk) reflex in patients with a moderately elevated magnesium level ( > 5 mEq/L). With the patient lying flat, support the knee in a moderately flexed position and tap the patellar tendon firmly just below the patella. Normally, the knee extends. An absent reflex suggests a magnesium level of 7 mEq/L or higher. Consult with the physician regarding significant changes.
3. Reassure the patient and significant others that altered mental functioning and muscle strength improve with treatment.
4. Keep the side rails up and the bed in its lowest position, with the wheels locked.
5. Assess the patient for the development of soft tissue calcification. Consult with the physician regarding significant findings.
6. Infants born to mothers receiving parenteral magnesium should be monitored for hypermagnesemia (e.g., neurologic depression, low Apgar scores).

7. Hypermagnesemia is often treated with IV calcium because it reverses the toxic effects of excess magnesium. The effects are temporary, and repeated doses may be necessary. Keep calcium at the bedside of symptomatic patients.

**Deficient knowledge** related to importance of avoiding excessive or inappropriate use of magnesium-containing medications, especially for patients with chronic renal failure.

**Desired outcome:** The patient verbalizes the importance of avoiding unusual magnesium intake and identifies potential sources of unwanted magnesium.

1. Caution patients with chronic renal failure to review all over-the-counter medications with the healthcare provider before use.
2. Provide a list of common magnesium-containing medications (see Box 11-2).
3. Patients with renal failure usually are on vitamin supplements. Caution these patients to avoid combination vitamin-mineral supplements because they usually contain magnesium.

## Patient-Family Teaching Guidelines

Give the patient and significant others verbal and written instructions for the following:

1. Medications: name, dosage, purpose, schedule, precautions, and potential side effects.
2. Indicators of hypermagnesemia. Review symptoms that require immediate medical attention: altered mental functioning, drowsiness, and muscle weakness.
3. Magnesium-containing medications that should be avoided (see Box 11-2).
4. The need to avoid magnesium-containing mineral supplements.

# Overview of Acid-Base Balance

## 12

For optimal functioning of the cells, metabolic processes maintain a steady balance between acids and bases. Arterial pH is an indirect measurement of hydrogen ion ($H^+$) concentration (i.e., the greater the concentration, the more acidic the solution and the lower the pH; the lower the concentration, the more alkaline the solution and the higher the pH). The pH is a reflection of the balance between carbon dioxide ($CO_2$), which is regulated by the lungs, and bicarbonate ($HCO_3^-$), a base regulated by the kidneys. $CO_2$ dissolves in solution to form carbonic acid ($H_2CO_3$), which is the key acid component in acid-base balance. Because $H_2CO_3$ is difficult to measure directly and $CO_2$ and $H_2CO_3$ are in balance, the acid component is expressed as $CO_2$ instead of $H_2CO_3$.

Normal acid-base ratio is 1:20, representing 1 part $CO_2$ (potential $H_2CO_3$) to 20 parts $HCO_3^-$. If this balance is altered, derangements in pH occur: if extra acids are present or there is a loss of base and the pH is less than 7.40, acidemia exists; if extra base is present or there is loss of acid and the pH is greater than 7.40, alkalemia is present. Several mechanisms regulate acid-base balance. These mechanisms are exceptionally sensitive to minute changes in pH. The body usually is able to maintain pH without outside intervention—if not at a normal level, at least within a life-sustaining range.

## Buffer System Responses
### Buffers

Buffers are present in all body fluids and act immediately (within 1 second) after an abnormal pH occurs. They combine with excess acid or base to form substances that do not affect pH. However, the effect of these buffers is limited.

1. **Bicarbonate:** The most important buffer, present in the largest quantity in body fluids. $HCO_3^-$ is generated by the kidneys and aids in the excretion of $H^+$.
2. **Phosphate:** Aids in the excretion of $H^+$ in the renal tubules.
3. **Ammonium ($NH_4^+$):** After an acid load, ammonia ($NH_3$) is produced by the renal tubular cell and is combined with $H^+$ in the renal tubule to form $NH_4^+$. This process allows greater renal excretion of $H^+$.
4. **Protein:** Present in cells, blood, and plasma. Hemoglobin is the most important protein buffer.

## Respiratory System

$H^+$ exerts direct action on the respiratory center in the brain. Acidemia increases alveolar ventilation to four to five times the normal level, whereas alkalemia decreases alveolar ventilation to 50% to 75% of the normal level. The response occurs quickly, within 1 to 2 minutes, during which time the lungs eliminate or retain $CO_2$ in direct relation to arterial pH. Although the respiratory system cannot correct imbalances completely, with healthy lungs, it is 50% to 70% effective.

## Renal System

The renal system regulates acid-base balance by increasing or decreasing $HCO_3^-$ concentration in body fluids. This is accomplished through a series of complex reactions that involve $H^+$, sodium ion ($Na^+$), and $HCO_3^-$ secretion, resorption, and conservation and $NH_3$ synthesis for excretion in the urine. $H^+$ secretion is regulated by the amount of $CO_2$ in extracellular fluid (ECF): the greater the concentration of $CO_2$, the greater the amount of $H^+$ secretion, resulting in acidic urine. When $H^+$ is excreted, $HCO_3^-$ is generated by the kidneys, helping maintain the 1:20 balance of acids and bases. When ECF is alkalotic, the kidneys conserve $H^+$ and eliminate $HCO_3^-$, resulting in alkalotic urine. Although the kidneys response to an abnormal pH is slow (several hours to days), healthy kidneys are usually able to adjust the imbalance to normal or near normal because of their ability to excrete large quantities of excess $HCO_3^-$ and $H^+$ from the body.

# Blood Gas Values

Blood gas analysis usually is based on arterial sampling. Venous values are given as a reference (Table 12-1).

## Arterial Blood Gas Analysis

Arterial blood gas (ABG) measurement is the best means of evaluating acid-base balance.

1. **pH:** Measures $H^+$ concentration to reflect acid-base status of the blood. Values reflect whether arterial pH is normal (7.40), acidic (< 7.40), or alkalotic (> 7.40). Because of the ability of compensatory mechanisms to "normalize" the pH, a near-normal value does not exclude the possibility of an acid-base disturbance.

2. **Partial pressure of $CO_2$ in arterial blood ($Paco_2$):** The respiratory component of acid-base regulation; adjusted by changes in the rate and depth of pulmonary ventilation. Hypercapnia ($Paco_2$ > 45 millimeters of mercury [mm Hg]) indicates alveolar hypoventilation and respiratory acidosis. Hyperventilation results in a $Paco_2$ less than 35 mm Hg and respiratory alkalosis in healthy lungs. Respiratory compensation occurs rapidly in metabolic acid-base disturbances. If any abnormality in $Paco_2$ exists, analysis of pH and $HCO_3^-$ parameters is important to determine whether the alteration in $Paco_2$ is the result of a primary respiratory disturbance or a compensatory response to a metabolic acid-base abnormality.

3. **$HCO_3^-$:** Serum $HCO_3^-$ is the major renal component of acid-base regulation. (It is reported as $CO_2$ content or total $CO_2$.) It is excreted or regenerated by the kidneys to maintain a normal acid-base environment. Decreased $HCO_3^-$ levels (< 24 milliequivalents/liter [mEq/L]) are indicative of metabolic acidosis (seen infrequently as a compensatory mechanism for respiratory alkalosis); elevated $HCO_3^-$ levels (> 28 mEq/L) reflect metabolic alkalosis, either as a primary metabolic disorder or as a compensatory alteration in response to respiratory acidosis.

4. **Base excess or deficit:** Indicates, in general terms, the amount of blood buffer (hemoglobin and plasma $HCO_3^-$) present. Abnormally high values reflect alkalosis; low values reflect acidosis. Normal value is ±2.

Table 12-1   Mixed venous blood gas values

| | Arterial Values | | Mixed Venous Values | |
| --- | --- | --- | --- | --- |
| | Perfect | Range | | |
| pH | 7.40 | 7.35-7.45 | pH | 7.33-7.43 |
| $Paco_2$ | 40 mm Hg | 35-45 mm Hg | $Pco_2$ | 41-51 mm Hg |
| $Pao_2$ | 95 mm Hg | 80-95 mm Hg | $Po_2$ | 35-49 mm Hg |
| Saturation | 95%-99% | | Saturation | 70%-75% |
| Base excess | ±2* | | | |
| Serum $HCO_3^-$ | 24 mEq/L | 22-26 mEq/L | $HCO_3^-$ | 24-28 mEq/L |

*Although serum $HCO_3^-$ is buffer, it is usually reported as total $CO_2$ or $CO_2$ content and not as serum $HCO_3^-$. Serum $HCO_3^-$ concentration is usually obtained separately from ABG analysis and is critical in determination of acid-base status. ($HCO_3^-$ reported with ABG results is usually calculated from pH and $Paco_2$.) Serum $HCO_3^-$ values should be obtained with initial ABG assessment and daily thereafter.

$Po_2$, Partial pressure of oxygen.

5. **Partial pressure of oxygen in arterial blood (Pao₂):** Has no primary role in acid-base regulation if it is within normal limits. The presence of hypoxemia with a $Pao_2$ less than 60 mm Hg can lead to anaerobic metabolism, resulting in lactic acid production and metabolic acidosis. Hypoxemia also may cause hyperventilation, resulting in respiratory alkalosis. There is a normal decline in $Pao_2$ in older adults.

6. **Saturation:** Measures the degree to which hemoglobin is saturated by oxygen ($O_2$). It can be affected by changes in temperature, pH, and $Paco_2$. When the $Pao_2$ falls below 60 mm Hg, there is a large drop in saturation. Pulse oximetry is often used for continuous $O_2$ saturation monitoring but is only accurate for saturation of more than 80% and is affected by decreased perfusion, vasoconstrictive agents, and nail polish.

## Step-by-Step Guide to Arterial Blood Gas Analysis

A systematic step-by-step analysis is critical to the accurate interpretation of ABG values. (For further information, see Tables 12-2, 12-3, and 12-4.)

1. **Step one:** Determine whether pH is normal. If it deviates from 7.40, note how much it deviates and in which direction. For example, pH higher than 7.40 indicates alkalemia; pH less than 7.40 indicates acidemia. Is the pH in the normal range of 7.35 to 7.45, or is it in the critical range of greater than 7.55 or less than 7.20?

2. **Step two:** Check the $Paco_2$. If it deviates from 40 mm Hg, how much does it deviate and in which direction? Does the change in $Paco_2$ correspond to the direction of the change in pH? The pH and $Paco_2$ should move in opposite directions. For example, as the $Paco_2$ increases, the pH should decrease (acidosis); as the $Paco_2$ decreases, the pH should increase (alkalosis).

3. **Step three:** Determine the $HCO_3^-$ value (may be referred to as $CO_2$ content or total $CO_2$). If it deviates from 24 mEq/L, note the degree and direction of deviation. Does the change in $HCO_3^-$ correspond to the change in pH? The $HCO_3^-$ and pH should move in the same direction. For example, if the $HCO_3^-$ decreases, the pH should decrease (acidosis); as the $HCO_3^-$ increases, the pH should increase (alkalosis).

Table 12-2  Arterial blood gas comparisons of acid-base disorders

|  |  | Alkalosis | | | Acidosis | | |
|---|---|---|---|---|---|---|---|
|  |  | $Paco_2$ | pH | $HCO_3^-$ | $Paco_2$ | pH | $HCO_3^-$ |
| Simple | Respiratory | 25 | 7.60* | 24 | 50 | 7.15* | 25 |
|  | Metabolic | 44 | 7.54 | 36 | 38 | 7.20 | 15 |
| Compensated | Respiratory | 25 | 7.54 | 21 | 66 | 7.37 | 34 |
|  | Metabolic | 50 | 7.42 | 31 | 23 | 7.28 | 9 |
| Mixed disorder |  | 40 | 7.56 | 38 | 50 | 7.20 | 20 |

*Note greater changes in pH with acute respiratory disorders because of delayed renal compensation.

Table 12-3  Quick assessment guide for acid-base imbalances

| Acid-Base Imbalance | pH | Paco$_2$ | HCO$_3^-$ | Clinical Signs and Symptoms | Common Causes |
|---|---|---|---|---|---|
| Acute respiratory acidosis | Decreased | Increased | No change | Tachycardia, tachypnea, diaphoresis, headache, restlessness, irritability, confusion, tremors, cyanosis, dysrhythmias, hypotension | Acute respiratory failure, cardiopulmonary disease, drug overdose, chest wall trauma, asphyxiation, CNS trauma/lesions, impaired muscles of respiration |
| Chronic respiratory acidosis (compensated) | Decreased | Increased | Increased* | Dyspnea; tachypnea; increase in CO$_2$ retention that exceeds compensatory ability; tremors, confusion, lethargy and somnolence, and coma | COPD, extreme obesity (pickwickian syndrome), superimposed infection on COPD |

*Continued*

**Table 12-3** Quick assessment guide for acid-base imbalances—cont'd

| Acid-Base Imbalance | pH | $Paco_2$ | $HCO_3^-$ | Clinical Signs and Symptoms | Common Causes |
|---|---|---|---|---|---|
| Acute respiratory alkalosis | Increased | Decreased | No change (decrease occurs if condition has been present for hours, providing that renal function is adequate) | Paresthesias, especially of fingers; dizziness | Hyperventilation, salicylate poisoning, hypoxemia (e.g., with pneumonia, pulmonary edema, pulmonary thromboembolism), gram-negative sepsis, CNS lesions, decreased lung compliance, inappropriate mechanical ventilation |
| Chronic respiratory alkalosis | Increased | Decreased | Decreased* | No symptoms | Hepatic failure, CNS lesions, pregnancy |

| | | | | | |
|---|---|---|---|---|---|
| Acute metabolic acidosis | Decreased | Decreased | Decreased | Tachypnea leading to Kussmaul's respirations, hypotension, cold and clammy skin, coma, and dysrhythmias | Shock, cardiopulmonary arrest (with resultant lactic acid production), ketoacidosis (e.g., diabetes, starvation, alcohol abuse), acute renal failure, ingestion of acids (e.g., salicylates), diarrhea |
| Chronic metabolic acidosis | Decreased | Decreased* (not as much as with acute metabolic acidosis) | Decreased | Fatigue, anorexia, malaise (may be related to chronic disease process and acidosis) | Chronic renal failure |
| Acute metabolic alkalosis | Increased | Increased* (can be as great as 60) | Increased | Muscular weakness and hyporeflexia (caused by severe hypokalemia), dysrhythmias, apathy, confusion, stupor | Volume depletion (Cl⁻ depletion) as result of vomiting, gastric drainage, diuretic use, or posthypercapnia; hyperadrenocorticism (e.g., Cushing's syndrome); aldosteronism; severe potassium depletion; excessive alkali intake |

*Continued*

Table 12-3    Quick assessment guide for acid-base imbalances—cont'd

| Acid-Base Imbalance | pH | $Pa_{CO_2}$ | $HCO_3^-$ | Clinical Signs and Symptoms | Common Causes |
|---|---|---|---|---|---|
| Chronic metabolic alkalosis | Increased | Increased* | Increased | Usually asymptomatic | Upper GI losses through continuous drainage; correction of hypercapnia if $Na^+$ and $K^+$ depletion remains uncorrected |

*Compensatory response.

*CNS*, Central nervous system; *Cl⁻*, chloride ion; *COPD*, chronic obstructive pulmonary disease; *GI*, gastrointestinal; *K⁺*, potassium ion.

Table 12-4  Acid-base rules: general guidelines

| Disturbance | Change in pH | Compensatory Response* | Results of Compensation |
|---|---|---|---|
| **Respiratory Acidosis** | | | |
| Acute | pH $\downarrow$ 0.08 for every 10 mm Hg $\uparrow$ in Paco$_2$ | Immediate release of tissue buffers (i.e., HCO$_3^-$) | 1 mEq/L $\uparrow$ in HCO$_3^-$ from patient's baseline for every 10 mm Hg $\uparrow$ in Paco$_2$ |
| Chronic | Depends on renal compensation; often near normal | $\uparrow$ Renal resorption of HCO$_3^-$; clinically evident after 8 hours; maximal effect in 3 to 5 days | 3.5 mEq/L $\uparrow$ in HCO$_3^-$ for every 10 mm Hg $\uparrow$ in Paco$_2$ |
| **Respiratory Alkalosis** | | | |
| Acute | pH $\uparrow$ 0.08 for every 10 mm Hg $\downarrow$ in Paco$_2$ | Immediate release of tissue buffers | 2 mEq/L $\downarrow$ in HCO$_3^-$ from patient's baseline for every 10 mm Hg $\downarrow$ in Paco$_2$ |
| Chronic | pH can be returned to normal if renal function is adequate | $\downarrow$ Renal resorption of HCO$_3^-$ | Maximal renal compensation causes HCO$_3^-$ to $\downarrow$ 5 mEq/L for every 10 mm Hg $\downarrow$ in Paco$_2$; maximal effect can take 7 to 9 days and may normalize pH |

*Compensatory responses in *healthy* lungs and kidneys.

*Continued*

Table 12-4   Acid-base rules: general guidelines—cont'd

| Disturbance | Change in pH | Compensatory Response* | Results of Compensation |
|---|---|---|---|
| **Metabolic Acidosis** | | | |
| Acute | pH $\downarrow$ 0.15 for every 10 mEq/L $\downarrow$ in $HCO_3^-$ | Hyperventilation occurs immediately | 1.2 mm Hg $\downarrow$ in $PaCO_2$ for every 1 mEq/L $\downarrow$ in $HCO_3^-$ |
| Chronic | pH is same as if no respiratory compensation were present | Hyperventilation | Effects of hyperventilation last only few days because $\downarrow$ in $PaCO_2$ causes further $\downarrow$ in renal resorption of $HCO_3^-$ |
| **Metabolic Alkalosis** | | | |
| Acute | pH $\uparrow$ 0.15 for every 10 mEq/L $\uparrow$ in $HCO_3^-$ | Hypoventilation occurs immediately | 0.7 mm Hg $\uparrow$ in $PaCO_2$ for every 1 mEq/L $\uparrow$ in $HCO_3^-$ |
| Chronic | pH is same as if respiratory compensation were present | Hypoventilation | Effects of hypoventilation last for only few days because $\uparrow$ in $PaCO_2$ causes $\uparrow$ renal excretion of $H^+$ and $\uparrow$ serum $HCO_3^-$ |

4. **Step four:** If both the $Paco_2$ and $HCO_3^-$ are abnormal, which value corresponds more closely to the pH value? For example, if the pH reflects acidemia, which value also reflects acidemia (an increased $Paco_2$ or a decreased $HCO_3^-$)? The value that more closely corresponds to the pH and deviates more from normal indicates the primary disturbance responsible for the alteration in pH. A mixed metabolic-respiratory disturbance or compensatory elements may be present when both $HCO_3^-$ and $Paco_2$ are abnormal.

5. **Step five:** Check $Pao_2$ and $O_2$ saturation to determine whether they are decreased, normal, or increased. Decreased $Pao_2$ and $O_2$ saturation can lead to lactic acidosis and may signal the need for increased concentrations of $O_2$. Conversely, high $Pao_2$ may be indicative of the need to decrease delivered concentrations of $O_2$.

## Mixed Venous Blood Gases

Mixed venous gases are usually obtained from a pulmonary artery catheter. (Blood from a central venous line may also be used if a pulmonary catheter is not present.) Mixed venous gases reflect acid-base status and oxygenation at the tissue level, thus providing information about tissue perfusion. ABGs give information about ventilatory function only.

## Arterial-Venous Difference

The difference between arterial $O_2$ content and venous $O_2$ content reflects the tissue extraction of $O_2$. ($O_2$ content is determined from $O_2$ saturation and hemoglobin). The normal value for arterial $O_2$ content is 18 milliliters (mL)/100 mL of blood, whereas the normal value for venous blood or pulmonary artery $O_2$ content is 14 mL/100 mL of blood. The difference between these two values increases when ventricular performance is impaired (e.g., right ventricular failure associated with congestive heart failure.

# Respiratory Acidosis

13

## Acute Respiratory Acidosis

Respiratory acidosis occurs as a result of alveolar hypoventilation and results in a carbon dioxide ($CO_2$) tension of arterial blood ($Paco_2$) greater than 40 millimeters of mercury (mm Hg; hypercapnia) and a pH less than 7.40. $Paco_2$ derangements are direct reflections of the degree of ventilatory dysfunction. Normally, $CO_2$ excretion equals $CO_2$ production. When an excess accumulation of $CO_2$ exists, the lungs fail to eliminate the necessary amounts to maintain the $Paco_2$ at 40 mm Hg. The degree to which the increased $Paco_2$ alters the pH depends on both the rapidity of onset and the body's ability to compensate through the blood buffer and renal systems. Although the blood buffer system acts immediately, it usually is not sufficient to maintain a normal pH in the presence of an elevated $Paco_2$. There is a delay (hours to days) before the effects of renal compensation can be noted. Therefore acute respiratory acidosis can have a profound effect on pH.

## Assessment

1. **Clinical manifestations:** Anxiety, restlessness, irritability, confusion, lethargy, psychosis with hallucinations, delusions, and delirium. (Stupor and coma are rare.)
2. **Physical assessment:** Increased heart rate (HR) and respiratory rate (RR), diaphoresis, and cyanosis. Severe hypercapnia may cause cerebral vasodilation, resulting in increased intracranial pressure (ICP) with papilledema. Another finding may be dilated conjunctival and facial blood vessels. (Central nervous system [CNS] depression leading to hypoventilation may result in a decreased RR.)
3. **Monitoring parameters:** Presence of ventricular dysrhythmias and increased ICP.

4. **History and risk factors (Box 13-1):**
   - *Acute respiratory disease:* Acute respiratory failure from a number of causes, including pneumonia, adult respiratory distress syndrome (ARDS), and acute exacerbation of underlying pulmonary dysfunction
   - *Overdose of drugs:* Oversedation with drugs that cause respiratory center depression
   - *Chest wall trauma*
     Flail chest
     Pneumothorax
   - *CNS trauma/lesions:* Can lead to depression of respiratory center
   - *Asphyxiation*
     Mechanical obstruction
     Anaphylaxis

---

**Box 13-1    Potential Causes of Acute Respiratory Acidosis**

**Pulmonary/Thoracic Disorders**

Severe pneumonia
Adult respiratory distress syndrome
Flail chest
Pneumothorax
Hemothorax
Smoke inhalation

**Increased Resistance to Air Flow**

Upper airway obstruction
Aspiration
Laryngospasm (e.g., anaphylaxis, severe hypocalcemia)
Severe bronchospasm
Severe, prolonged acute asthma attack

**Central Nervous System Depression**

Sedative overdose
Anesthesia
Cerebral trauma
Cerebral infarct

*Continued*

> ### Box 13-1    Potential Causes of Acute Respiratory Acidosis—cont'd
>
> **Metabolic Causes**
> High-carbohydrate diet
>
> **Neuromuscular Abnormalities**
> Guillain-Barré syndrome
> Myasthenia gravis crisis
> Hypokalemia
> High cervical cordotomy
> Drugs (e.g., curare, aminoglycosides)
> Toxins
> Hypophosphatemia
>
> **Systemic Causes**
> Cardiac arrest
> Massive pulmonary embolus
> Severe pulmonary edema
>
> **Mechanical Ventilation**
> Fixed minute ventilation with increased $CO_2$ production
> Inappropriate dead space
> Equipment failure

- *Impaired respiratory muscles*
  Hypokalemia
  Guillain-Barré syndrome
  Myasthenia gravis crisis
- *Iatrogenic*
  Inappropriate mechanical ventilation (e.g., increased dead space, insufficient rate or volume). Low tidal volumes may be used to minimize lung injury in patients with ARDS leading to a *permissive hypercapnia*. (The $Paco_2$ is allowed to slowly increase to 60 to 70 mm Hg.) High fraction of inspired oxygen ($Fio_2$) in the presence of chronic $CO_2$ retention.

## Diagnostic Tests

1. **Arterial blood gas (ABG) analysis:** Aids in diagnosis and determination of severity of respiratory acidosis. $Paco_2$ is

greater than 40 mm Hg, and pH is less than 7.40. All individuals with elevated $Paco_2$ have some degree of hypoxemia with breathing room air. The hypoxemia is usually present first and is initially more pronounced than the hypercapnia. A small increase in $Paco_2$ indicates severe pulmonary dysfunction.

2. **Total CO$_2$:** Reflects metabolic and base balance. Initially, bicarbonate ion ($HCO_3^-$) values are normal (24 to 28 milliequivalents/liter [mEq/L]) unless a mixed disorder is present.

3. **Serum electrolytes:** Usually not altered, depending on the etiology of respiratory acidosis.

4. **Chest radiograph:** Determines the presence of underlying respiratory disease.

5. **Drug screen:** Determines the presence and quantity of drug if an overdose is suspected.

## Collaborative Management

1. **Restoration of normal acid-base balance:** Accomplished with supporting respiratory function. If $Paco_2$ is greater than 50 to 60 mm Hg and clinical signs such as cyanosis and lethargy are present, the patient usually needs intubation and mechanical ventilation. Generally, use of sodium bicarbonate ($NaHCO_3$) is avoided because of the risk of metabolic alkalosis when the respiratory disturbance has been corrected. In patients with severe acidemia (pH < 7.20), small doses of $NaHCO_3$ (44 to 88 mEq) may be given as an infusion over 5 to 10 minutes; recheck total $CO_2$ 30 minutes after infusion to assess effect. ($NaHCO_3$ should be avoided in patients with pulmonary edema.) Although a life-threatening pH must be promptly corrected to an acceptable level, a normal pH is not the immediate goal.

2. **Treatment of the underlying disorder**

## Nursing Diagnoses and Interventions

**Impaired gas exchange** related to alveolar hypoventilation from underlying disease process.

**Desired outcome:** The patient has adequate oxygen supply and alveolar ventilation as evidenced by an oxygen tension of arterial blood ($Pao_2$) of 60 mm Hg or higher, $Paco_2$ of 45 mm Hg or lower, pH of 7.35 to 7.45, RR of 12 to 20 breaths/minute with a normal pattern and depth (eupnea), and absence of adventitious breath sounds; impairment of mental status and restlessness are reduced or absent.

1. Monitor serial ABG results to detect the continued presence of hypercapnia or hypoxemia. Report significant findings (e.g., variances of 10 to 20 mm Hg in $Paco_2$ or $Pao_2$).

2. Assess and document the character of respiratory effort: rate, depth, rhythm, and use of accessory muscles of respiration.

3. Assess the patient for signs and symptoms of respiratory distress: restlessness, anxiety, confusion, and tachypnea (RR > 20 breaths/minute).

4. Position the patient for comfort and to ensure optimal gas exchange. Usually, a semi-Fowler's position allows for adequate expansion of the chest wall, but the specific pathologic process must be considered in the positioning of patients.

   - For unilateral lung disease in a patient with mechanical ventilation, a side-lying (lateral decubitus) position may increase perfusion in the dependent (healthy) lung and increase ventilation to the upper (diseased) lung ("good side down" position).

   - For patients with ARDS who need mechanical ventilation, the prone position may improve gas exchange with an average increase in $Pao_2$ of 20 to 60 mm Hg, especially if instituted in the early phases of the lung injury. Increased gas exchange results from improving the ventilation-perfusion mismatch by increasing perfusion of the dorsal aspect of the lung tissue and decreasing the shunt. (Perfusion is greater in the dorsal aspect of the lung independent of the patient's position.) The improved gas exchange often leads to a reduction in $Fio_2$ and positive end expiratory pressure, further protecting the lung from injury. Other benefits of this positioning include downward shifting of the diaphragm, mobilization of pulmonary secretions, and improved lymphatic drainage, all contributing to improved pulmonary dynamics. Many patients with ARDS benefit from the prone position, and a brief trial (30 minutes) in this position is recommended to identify patients who respond favorably. Patients may be maintained in the prone position until pulmonary function has improved. The time patients can tolerate the prone position and the respiratory benefits vary and must be determined on an individual basis. Improved ventilatory status is noted by improvement in breath sounds and ABG values (increased $Pao_2$ on the same or less oxygen concentration and ventilator settings). A prone position may be contraindicated in the following cases: spinal instability, increased ICP, multiple trauma, extreme obesity, and abdominal surgery.

5. Remove secretions by encouraging coughing or by suctioning. Prone positioning can also enhance postural drainage and clearance of secretions.

6. If ordered, monitor mechanical ventilation: ventilator settings, endotracheal and tracheal tube function, ventilator and breathing circuit function, and peak airway pressure.

7. Monitor for the presence of bowel sounds and distension to prevent a decrease in diaphragmatic movement from abdominal pressure. (Gastoparesis can occur as the result of changes in gastric rhythm and tone.)

**Acute confusion** related to disturbance in acid-base regulation.

**Desired outcome:** The patient verbalizes orientation to person, place, and time and does not exhibit evidence of injury caused by confusion.

1. Monitor ABG and serum $CO_2$ results. Notify the physician regarding abnormal values and significant changes (e.g., variances of 10 to 20 mm Hg in $Paco_2$ and $Pao_2$). At frequent intervals, assess and document the patient's level of consciousness (LOC) and orientation to person, place, and time.

2. Use reality therapy, such as familiar photos, a calendar, and a clock with a face that is large enough for the patient to see. Keep these items at the bedside and within the patient's visual field.

3. Keep the bed in its lowest position, with all side rails up and the wheels locked.

4. If the patient is allowed out of bed, remind the patient to ask for assistance before getting up.

5. Offer confused patients the opportunity to toilet at frequent intervals. Many falls result from disoriented or unsteady patients' attempts to toilet.

6. Use a night light to minimize confusion in an unfamiliar and unlit environment.

7. If the patient's confusion persists despite reorientation, increase the frequency of observations, with concomitant reorientation and documentation. Alert the physician to continued or increasing confusion.

8. Reassure the patient and significant others that the patient's confusion abates with treatment.

9. If the patient remains at risk for injury, obtain a prescription for a protective restraining device, per agency policy.
   - Document the need for a restraining device on the basis of the patient's behavior on initiation and every 8 hours thereafter.
   - Choose the least restrictive device that protects the patient. Add additional devices as needed, based on documented patient behaviors.
   - Document the type of device used. A protective vest is applied to the upper torso with the crisscross or V in the front. Soft limb protectors are applied to the upper extremities (may be applied to upper and lower extremities in some cases).
   - Monitor the patient every 15 to 30 minutes while restraints are in use, documenting mental status and response to protective devices.
   - Document the frequency (at least every 2 hours) of device removal, repositioning of patient, and reapplication of the device.

**Impaired oral mucous membrane** related to abnormal breathing pattern.

**Desired outcome:** Absence of oral inflammation and infection.

1. Assess the patient's oral mucous membrane, lips, and tongue every 2 hours, noting the presence of dryness, exudate, swelling, blisters, and ulcers.

2. If the patient is alert and able to take fluids orally, offer frequent sips of water or ice chips to alleviate dryness.

3. Perform mouth care every 2 to 4 hours, with a soft-bristled toothbrush to cleanse the teeth and a moistened cloth or toothette (small sponge on a stick) to moisten crusty areas or exudate on the tongue and oral mucosa. If the patient is intubated, suction the mouth to remove fluid and debris.

4. If indicated, use an artificial saliva preparation to assist in keeping the mucous membrane moist. Avoid the use of lemon and glycerine swabs, which can contribute to dryness.

5. Apply vitamin A and D ointment in a lanolin-petrolatum base lip balm to keep lips from drying and aid in healing cracked lips.

**Disturbed sleep pattern** related to frequent treatments and procedures.

**Desired outcome:** The patient sleeps undisturbed for at least 90 minutes at a time and relates a feeling of being rested.

1. Gather information about the patient's normal sleep habits: bedtime rituals; usual position; hours of sleep required; number of pillows used; and sensitivity to light, noise, and touch. Based on the data gathered, attempt to incorporate the patient's needs into the care plan.
2. Cluster activities and procedures to minimize the need for interrupting the patient's sleep. Even brief (30-second) interruptions of sleep can result in feelings of fatigue.
3. Attempt to administer unpleasant or uncomfortable procedures or treatments at least 1 hour before bedtime to allow time for relaxation before the patient attempts to sleep.
4. Offer backrubs, repositioning, and relaxation techniques (e.g., quiet music, instructions for imagery) at bedtime.
5. If the patient requires a daytime nap because of fatigue, provide opportunities to sleep between 1 PM and 3 PM. Sleep attained at this time is most restful and least likely to disrupt nighttime sleep. Discourage napping after 7 PM; it may prevent the patient from falling asleep and maintaining a normal sleep cycle.
6. Monitor the level of daytime alertness and daytime functioning.

**Ineffective family coping** related to stress reaction from catastrophic illness of family member.

**Desired outcome:** Family members exhibit improved coping mechanisms, seek support from others, and discuss concerns among the family unit.

1. Establish an open line of communication with the family, providing an atmosphere in which family members can ask questions, ventilate feelings, and discuss concerns among other family members.
2. Assess family members' knowledge about the patient's therapies and treatments. Provide information as needed and reinforce information the family has received from other healthcare members.

3. Provide opportunities and areas for family members to talk privately and share concerns with healthcare members.
4. Determine effective coping strategies that have been used by the family in other stressful situations. Support and encourage the family to continue the use of healthy, effective coping strategies.
5. Enable family members to spend time alone with the patient for short, frequent intervals.
6. Encourage family members to pursue diversion activities outside the hospital to help alleviate the stress of the immediate situation. Families often feel the need for "permission" from healthcare members to leave the waiting room or hospital.
7. Offer realistic hope.

# Chronic Respiratory Acidosis

Chronic respiratory acidosis is a disorder that occurs in pulmonary diseases (e.g., chronic emphysema, bronchitis) in which effective alveolar ventilation is decreased and a ventilation-perfusion mismatch is present. In addition to the impaired ventilatory mechanisms, the central respiratory drive is also reduced, inherently or coexisting with metabolic alkalosis from steroids or diuretics. Chronic hypercapnia also can occur with obesity because of the added weight on the rib cage and abdomen decreasing lung compliance. In patients with chronic lung disease, a nearly normal pH can be seen if renal function is normal, even if the $Paco_2$ is as high as 60 mm Hg; chronic compensatory metabolic alkalosis (serum $HCO_3^- > 28$ mEq/L) occurs and maintains an acceptable acid-base environment, which results in compensated respiratory acidosis and a normal or near normal pH. Patients with chronic lung disease can have acute rises in $Paco_2$ from superimposed disease states such as pneumonia. If the chronic compensatory mechanisms in place (e.g., elevated $HCO_3^-$) are inadequate to meet the sudden increase in $Paco_2$, decompensation may occur with a resultant decrease in pH.

## Assessment

1. **Clinical manifestations:** If the $Paco_2$ does not exceed the body's ability to compensate, no specific findings are noted.

If $Pa_{CO_2}$ rises rapidly, the following may occur: dull head-ache, weakness, dyspnea, asterixis, agitation, and insomnia progressing to somnolence and coma.

2. **Physical assessment:** Tachypnea and cyanosis. Severe hypercapnia ($Pa_{CO_2} > 70$ mm Hg) may cause cerebral vaso-dilation, resulting in increased ICP, papilledema, and dilated conjunctival and facial blood vessels. Depending on the underlying pathophysiology, edema may be present from right ventricular failure.

3. **History and risk factors (Box 13-2):**
   - *Chronic obstructive pulmonary disease (COPD)*
     Emphysema
     Bronchitis
   - *Extreme obesity*
     Pickwickian syndrome
   - *Development of superimposed acute respiratory infection in a patient with COPD*
   - *Exposure to pulmonary toxins*
     Occupational risk
     Pollution

## Diagnostic Tests

1. **ABG values:** Provide data necessary for determining the diagnosis and severity of respiratory acidosis. Although the $Pa_{CO_2}$ is elevated, the pH is on the acidic (low) side of normal because of renal compensation, except in patients with acute pulmonary infection. If the $Pa_{CO_2}$ has increased abruptly from the baseline value, a pH lower than normal may be seen.

2. **Total $CO_2$:** Serum $CO_2$ (equivalent to $HCO_3^-$) is espe-cially helpful in determining the level of metabolic com-pensation that has occurred (e.g., increased $HCO_3^-$ with a near normal pH if fully compensated). This information is particularly useful in identifying "mixed" acid-base dis-turbances (see Chapter 17) because the $HCO_3^-$ is expected to be elevated in chronic respiratory acidosis. If the $HCO_3^-$ is normal or low, this could be diagnostic of a pathologic process concurrent with the respiratory acidosis (e.g., meta-bolic acidosis).

3. **Chest radiograph:** Determines the extent of underlying pulmonary disease and identifies further pathologic changes

---

### Box 13-2    Potential Causes of Chronic Respiratory Acidosis

---

**Obstructive Diseases**

Emphysema
Chronic bronchitis
Cystic fibrosis
Obstructive sleep apnea

**Restriction of Ventilation**

Kyphoscoliosis
Hydrothorax
Severe chronic pneumonitis
Obesity-hypoventilation (pickwickian) syndrome

**Neuromuscular Abnormalities**

Spinal cord injuries
Poliomyelitis
Muscular dystrophy
Multiple sclerosis
Amyotrophic lateral sclerosis
Diaphragmatic paralysis
Myxedema

**Depression of the Respiratory Center**

Brain tumor
Bulbar poliomyelitis
Chronic sedative overdose
Central sleep apnea

---

that may be responsible for acute exacerbation (e.g., pneumonia).

4. **Electrocardiogram (ECG):** Identifies cardiac involvement from COPD. For example, right-sided heart failure is a complication of chronic bronchitis.

5. **Sputum culture:** Determines the presence of pathogens causing an acute exacerbation of a chronic pulmonary disease (e.g., pneumonia), present in patients with COPD.

## Collaborative Management

1. **Oxygen therapy:** Used cautiously (i.e., at a rate not usually > 3 L/minute) in patients with chronic $CO_2$ retention for whom hypoxemia, rather than hypercapnia, stimulates ventilation. The patient may need intubation and mechanical ventilation for stupor and coma precipitated by oxygen if the drive to breathe is eliminated by high concentrations of oxygen.
2. **Pharmacotherapy:** Bronchodilators and antibiotics, as indicated. Narcotics and sedatives can depress the respiratory center and are avoided unless the patient has intubation and mechanical ventilation. Progesterone may be given as a respiratory stimulant; it may be especially beneficial to obese patients.
3. **Intravenous (IV) fluids:** Maintain adequate hydration for mobilizing pulmonary secretions.
4. **Chest physiotherapy:** Aids in expectoration of sputum; includes postural drainage if hypersecretions are present. Assess the patient closely during this procedure because it may be poorly tolerated, especially the postural drainage component.

## Nursing Diagnoses and Interventions

**Impaired gas exchange** related to trapping of $CO_2$ from pulmonary tissue destruction (appropriate for the patient with COPD).

**Desired outcome:** ABG values reflect a $Pa_{CO_2}$ and pH within an acceptable range based on the patient's underlying pulmonary disease. Impairment of mental status or restlessness is absent or reduced.

1. Monitor serial ABG results to assess the patient's response to therapy. Report significant findings to the physician: increasing $Pa_{CO_2}$ and decreasing pH. ABGs drawn while patient is sleeping may show an increased $Pa_{CO_2}$ from a further decrease in central respiratory drive. Assess for nocturnal hypercapnia; cerebral dilatation from increased $Pa_{CO_2}$ can cause morning headaches, daytime somnolence, confusion, intellectual impairment, and decreased sleep quality.

2. Assess and document the patient's respiratory status: RR and rhythm, exertional effort, and breath sounds. Compare pretreatment findings with posttreatment (e.g., oxygen therapy, physiotherapy, or medications) findings for evidence of improvement.

3. Assess and document the patient's LOC. If $Paco_2$ increases, be alert to subtle, progressive changes in mental status. A common progression is *agitation → insomnia → somnolence → coma*. To avoid a comatose state secondary to rising $CO_2$ levels, always evaluate the arousability of a patient with an elevated $Paco_2$ who appears to be sleeping. Notify the physician if the patient is difficult to arouse.

4. Ensure appropriate delivery of prescribed oxygen therapy. Assess the patient's respiratory status after every change in $Fio_2$. Patients with chronic $CO_2$ retention may be sensitive to increases in $Fio_2$, resulting in depressed ventilatory drive. If the patient needs mechanical ventilation, be aware of the importance of maintaining the compensated acid-base environment. If the $Paco_2$ was decreased too rapidly by a high RR delivered by mechanical ventilation, a severe metabolic alkalosis could develop, resulting in severe neurologic abnormalities (e.g., seizures, coma). The sudden onset of metabolic alkalosis may also lead to hypocalcemia, which can result in tetany (see Chapter 9).

5. Assess for the presence of bowel sounds and monitor for gastric distention, which can impede movement of the diaphragm and restrict ventilatory effort further.

6. Assess diet; diets rich in carbohydrates yield a greater $CO_2$ load, which may compromise patients with limited ventilatory reserve or respiratory failure.

7. If the patient is not intubated, encourage the use of pursed-lip breathing (inhalation through the nose, with slow exhalation through pursed lips), which helps airways remain open and allows for better air excursion. Optimally, this technique diminishes air entrapment in the lungs and makes respiratory effort more efficient.

**Ineffective airway clearance** related to viscous secretions and fatigue.

**Desired outcome:** Auscultation of the patient's airway reveals the absence of adventitious breath sounds.

1. Be alert to increased fatigue or lethargy as a potential sign of increasing $Paco_2$.

2. If the patient is unable to raise secretions independently, perform suctioning as often as is determined with assessment findings.

3. If prescribed, administer chest physiotherapy. (Chest physiotherapy may be contraindicated in some patients with chronic $CO_2$ retention.) Evaluate the effectiveness of therapy by assessing breath sounds, ABG results, and patency of the airway both before and after treatment.

4. Ensure adequate fluid intake to compensate for increased insensible losses caused by increased RR, febrile state, and diaphoresis. Adequate hydration makes secretions less viscous and easier to mobilize.

5. Encourage the nonintubated patient to continue pursed-lip breathing (inhalation through the nose, with slow exhalation through pursed lips), which increases the efficiency and effectiveness of respiratory effort.

(For other nursing diagnoses and interventions, see the section on Acute Respiratory Acidosis for the following: "Impaired oral mucous membrane related to abnormal breathing pattern" [see pp. 180-181] and "Disturbed sleep pattern related to frequent treatments and procedures" [see p. 181].)

# Respiratory Alkalosis 14

## Acute Respiratory Alkalosis

Respiratory alkalosis occurs as a result of an increase in the rate of alveolar ventilation (alveolar hyperventilation). It is defined by a partial pressure of carbon dioxide in arterial blood ($Pa_{CO_2}$) less than 40 millimeters of mercury (mm Hg; hypocapnia) and a pH greater than 7.40. Acute alveolar hyperventilation most frequently is the result of anxiety and is commonly referred to as *hyperventilation syndrome*. In addition, numerous physiologic disorders (see the subsequent History and Risk Factors) can cause acute hypocapnia, which results in increased pH. (Hypocapnia is the most common acid-base disturbance in critically ill patients.) The rise in pH is modified to a small degree by intracellular buffering. To compensate for increased carbon dioxide ($CO_2$) loss and the resultant base excess, hydrogen ions ($H^+$) are released from tissue buffers, which in turn lower plasma bicarbonate ($HCO_3^-$) concentration (a reduction of ~2 milliequivalents [mEq]/liter [L]/10 mm Hg decrease in the $Pa_{CO_2}$). The kidneys' response to respiratory alkalosis is slow (several hours to days); thus acute respiratory alkalosis is usually resolved before renal compensation can occur.

### Assessment

1. **Clinical manifestations:** Dizziness, vertigo, anxiety, euphoria, paresthesias, palpitations, and circumoral numbness. Chest pain from cardiac and noncardiac causes is common. Nausea and vomiting may be present. In extreme alkalosis, confusion, tetany, syncope, and seizures may occur.
2. **Physical assessment:** Increased rate and depth of respirations.

3. **Electrocardiogram (ECG) findings:** Cardiac dysrhythmias.
4. **History and risk factors (Box 14-1):**
   - *Anxiety:* The patient is often unaware of hyperventilation.
   - *Acute hypoxemia:* Pulmonary disorders (e.g., pneumonia, mild to moderate asthmatic attack, pulmonary edema, pulmonary thromboembolism) cause hypoxemia, which stimulates the ventilatory effort in the initial stages of the disease process.

---

### Box 14-1   Potential Causes of Acute Respiratory Alkalosis

Hypoxemia

Pneumonia
Hypotension
Severe anemia
Congestive heart failure
High altitude (> 6500 ft)

Stimulation of Pulmonary or Pleural Receptors

Pulmonary emboli
Pulmonary edema
Asthma
Inhalation of irritants
Interstitial fibrosis

Central (Direct) Stimulation of the Respiratory Center

Anxiety
Pain
Drugs (salicylates, catecholamines, theophylline)
Intracerebral trauma (increased intracranial pressure)
Acute cerebral vascular accident (unexplained
   respiratory alkalosis is a poor prognostic sign)

Hyperventilation—Mechanical or Psychogenic Metabolic

Fever
Sepsis (gram negative)
Hepatic disease
Hormonal (progesterone)

---

- *Metabolic states*
  Fever and sepsis, especially gram-negative–induced septicemia (respiratory alkalosis is an important early finding in septicemia), hepatic disease, and hormones (progestin).
- *Salicylate intoxication*
- *Excessive mechanical ventilation*
- *Central nervous system (CNS) trauma:* Strokes, tumors, and trauma may result in damage to the respiratory center.

## Diagnostic Tests

1. **Arterial blood gas (ABG) values:** $Paco_2$ less than 40 mm Hg and pH greater than 7.40 are present. A decreased oxygen tension of arterial blood ($Pao_2$), along with the clinical picture (e.g., pneumonia, pulmonary edema, pulmonary embolism), may help diagnose the etiology of the respiratory alkalosis. In patients breathing spontaneously, a $Paco_2$ less than 20 to 25 mm Hg may indicate a poor prognosis.
2. **Serum electrolytes:** Determine the presence of metabolic acid-base disorders. A $HCO_3^-$ concentration greater or less than a reduction of 2 mEq/L/10 mm Hg decrease in $Pco_2$ indicates a mixed acid-base imbalance (e.g., a metabolic alkalosis or acidosis). Hyperkalemia is seen initially. Prolonged respiratory alkalosis can lead to hypokalemia.
3. **Serum phosphate:** May fall to less than 0.5 milligrams/deciliter (mg/dL; normal is 3 to 4.5 mg/dL) because of the alkalosis, which causes increased uptake of phosphate by the cells.
4. **Lactic acidosis:** Moderate increase in lactic acid is seen.
5. **ECG:** Detects cardiac dysrhythmias, which may be present with alkalosis.

## Collaborative Management

1. **Treatment of the underlying disorder**
2. **Reassurance:** If anxiety is the cause of the decreased $Paco_2$. For severe symptoms, it may be necessary for the patient to rebreathe into a paper bag (this increases the $Pco_2$ in the inspired air). Instead of a paper bag, an oxygen mask with an attached $CO_2$ reservoir may be prescribed. It is important to recheck arterial pH to ensure metabolic acidosis does not occur from the decrease in $HCO_3^-$ as the $Pco_2$ returns to normal.

3. **Oxygen therapy:** If hypoxemia is the causative factor.
4. **Adjustments to mechanical ventilators:** Settings are checked and adjustments made to ventilatory parameters in response to ABG results that signal hypocapnia. Respiratory rate (RR) or volume is decreased, and dead space is added, if necessary.
5. **Pharmacotherapy:** Sedatives and tranquilizers may be given for anxiety-induced respiratory alkalosis.

## Nursing Diagnoses and Interventions

**Ineffective breathing pattern** related to hyperventilation from anxiety.

**Desired outcome:** The patient's breathing pattern is effective as evidenced by a $Paco_2$ of at least 35 mm Hg and a pH of 7.45 or lower.

1. To help alleviate anxiety, reassure the patient that a staff member will remain with the patient.
2. Encourage the patient to breathe slowly. Pace the patient's breathing by having the patient mimic your own breathing pattern.
3. Monitor the patient's cardiac rhythm, notifying the physician if dysrhythmias occur. With acute respiratory alkalosis, even a modest alkalosis can precipitate dysrhythmias in a patient with a preexisting heart disease who is also taking cardiotropic drugs.
4. Administer sedatives or tranquilizers as prescribed.
5. Have the patient rebreathe into a paper bag or an oxygen mask with an attached $CO_2$ reservoir, if prescribed.
6. Ensure that the patient rests undisturbed after the breathing pattern has stabilized. Hyperventilation can result in fatigue.

NOTE: Hyperventilation may lead to hypocalcemic tetany despite a normal or near normal calcium level because of increased binding of calcium (see Chapter 9).

## Chronic Respiratory Alkalosis

This is a state of chronic hypocapnia, which stimulates the renal compensatory response and results in a greater decrease in plasma $HCO_3^-$ (a reduction of 4 mEq/L/10 mm Hg in $Pco_2$). Maximal renal compensatory response requires 2 to 4 days to occur.

## Assessment

1. **Clinical manifestations:** Individuals with chronic respiratory alkalosis usually are asymptomatic.
2. **Physical assessment:** Increased RR and depth.
3. **History and risk factors:**
   - *Cerebral disease*
     Tumor
     Encephalitis
   - *Chronic hepatic insufficiency*
   - *Pregnancy, hormone replacement therapy*
   - *Chronic hypoxemia*
     Adaptation to high altitude, cyanotic heart disease, and lung disease resulting in decreased compliance (e.g., fibrosis)

## Diagnostic Tests

1. **ABG values:** $Paco_2$ is less than 35 mm Hg, with a nearly normal pH; $Pao_2$ may be decreased if hypoxemia is the causative factor.
2. **Serum electrolytes:** Probably is normal with the exception of total $CO_2$ (serum $HCO_3^-$), which decreases as renal compensation occurs. Maximal renal compensation takes 7 to 9 days with normalization of pH.
3. **Phosphate levels:** Hypophosphatemia (as low as 0.5 mg/dL) may be seen with intense hyperventilation. Alkalosis causes increased uptake of phosphate by the cells.

## Collaborative Management

1. **Treatment of the underlying cause**
2. **Oxygen therapy:** If hypoxemia is present and identified as a causative factor in respiratory alkalosis.

## Nursing Diagnoses and Interventions

Nursing diagnoses and interventions are specific to the pathophysiologic process.

# Metabolic Acidosis

15

## Acute Metabolic Acidosis

Metabolic acidosis is caused by a primary decrease in plasma bicarbonate, as reflected by a serum bicarbonate of less than 24 milliequivalents/liter (mEq/L) with a pH less than 7.40. The decrease in serum bicarbonate is caused by one of the following mechanisms: 1, increase in the concentration of hydrogen ions ($H^+$) in the form of nonvolatile acids (e.g., ketoacidosis associated with diabetes and alcoholism; lactic acidosis); 2, loss of alkali (e.g., severe diarrhea, intestinal malabsorption); or 3, decreased acid excretion by the kidneys (e.g., acute and chronic renal failure). The decrease in pH stimulates respirations. The body's attempts to compensate occur rapidly, as manifested by lowering of the partial pressure of carbon dioxide in arterial blood ($Paco_2$), which may be reduced by as much as 10 to 15 millimeters of mercury (mm Hg). The most important mechanism for ridding the body of excess $H^+$ is the increase in acid excretion by the kidneys. However, nonvolatile acids may accumulate more rapidly than they can be neutralized by the body's buffers, compensated for by the respiratory system, or excreted by the kidneys. (Box 15-1 describes the classification of acidosis.)

## Assessment

1. **Clinical manifestations:** Findings vary, depending on the underlying disease states and severity of the acid-base disturbance. Headache, nausea, vomiting, and diarrhea may be present. There may be changes in the level of consciousness, ranging from fatigue and confusion to stupor and coma.

2. **Physical assessment:** Decreased blood pressure; tachypnea leading to alveolar hyperventilation, which may progress to

Kussmaul's respirations; cold and clammy skin; presence of dysrhythmias; and shock state.

3. **History and risk factors** (see Box 15-1):
   - *Renal disease*
     Acute renal failure
     Renal tubular acidosis (RTA)
   - *Loss of alkali*
     Draining wounds (e.g., pancreatic fistulas)

---

**Box 15-1    Acidosis Classification and Potential Causes of Metabolic Acidosis**

| Normal Anion Gap (12 [±2] mEq/L) | High Anion Gap (>14 mEq/L) |
|---|---|
| **Gastrointestinal Causes (Loss of $HCO_3^-$)** | **Metabolic Causes** |
| 1. Diarrhea | 1. Lactic Acidosis |
| 2. Biliary and pancreatic drainage |   ■ Type A: tissue hypoxia (e.g., shock, heart failure, sepsis) |
| 3. Urethral sigmoidostomy or ileostomy |   ■ Type B: hypoglycemia, diabetes mellitus, hepatic failure, ethanol, salicylates, and malignant diseases |
| 4. Cholestyramine | 2. Ketoacidosis |
| **Renal Causes (renal tubular acidosis [RTA])** |   ■ Diabetes mellitus |
| 1. Type 1: distal RTA (associated with autoimmune disease) |   ■ Alcoholism |
| 2. Type 2: proximal RTA (caused by carbonic anhydrase inhibitors [e.g., Diamox]) |   ■ Starvation |
| 3. Type 4: hyperkalemic RTA (associated with diabetes and adrenal cortex disorders)* | **Renal Causes** |
|  | 1. Renal failure (acute or chronic) |
| 4. Renal insufficiency or early renal failure | **Exogenous Causes** |
|  | 1. Methanol |
|  | 2. Salicylates |
|  | 3. Ethylene glycol |

*Most common form of RTA in adults.

Diarrhea
Ureterostomy
Cholestyramine
- *Ketoacidosis*
Diabetes mellitus (DM)
Alcoholism: more common in women who binge drink
Starvation
- *Lactic acidosis:* Respiratory or circulatory failure, drugs and toxins, septic shock, and hereditary disorders; can be associated with other disease states such as leukemia, solid tumors, pancreatitis, bacterial infection, and uncontrolled DM
- *Poisoning and drug toxicity*
Salicylates
Methanol
Ethylene glycol
Ammonium chloride
Cocaine
Ecstacy
Methamphetamine: may be seen in trauma patients who use methamphetamine

## Diagnostic Tests

1. **Arterial blood gas (ABG) values:** The pH ($<7.40$) and degree of respiratory compensation as reflected by $Paco_2$, which usually is less than 35 mm Hg, should be determined. (To estimate the degree of anticipated respiratory compensation, add 15 to the serum $HCO_3^-$ level.) Increasing levels of carbon dioxide ($CO_2$) at the tissue level may not be reflected in ABGs, although the overall $CO_2$ elimination is decreased (see the next point).

2. **Mixed venous blood gases:** Mixed venous $CO_2$ is markedly higher than arterial $Pco_2$. The higher $CO_2$ is not related to impaired pulmonary function; it is the result of the generation and accumulation of $CO_2$ at the cellular level during shock states, congestive heart failure, and cardiac arrest. Mixed venous gases should be obtained simultaneously with ABGs.

3. **Total $CO_2$:** Total $CO_2$ determines the presence of metabolic acidosis (bicarbonate ion [$HCO_3^-$] $<24$ mEq/L).

4. **Serum electrolytes:** Elevated potassium may be present because of the exchange of intracellular potassium for $H^+$ during the body's attempt to normalize the acid-base environment. Elevated $Cl^-$ is a common finding.

   ■ *Anion gap:* In an attempt to identify the cause of metabolic acidosis, an analysis of serum electrolytes to detect anion gap may be helpful. Anion gap reflects unmeasurable anions present in plasma and is calculated by subtracting the sum of chloride and bicarbonate from the plasma sodium concentration. An increase in anion gap is present with diabetic ketoacidosis (DKA), lactic acidosis, and other states in which nonvolatile acids accumulate. Nonvolatile acids can be either organic acids (e.g., lactate, ketones) or inorganic acids (e.g., salicylate, formic acid [from methanol ingestion]). Organic acids can be converted to $HCO_3^-$ by the liver. If the acids are produced or accumulate more rapidly than the liver can metabolize them, acidosis occurs. With treatment of the underlying disorder, the organic acids still present in the body are converted to $HCO_3^-$. (Ketones that have been spilled in the urine are not available for this conversion to $HCO_3^-$.) High anion gap acidosis (>14 mEg/L) can be the result of an accumulation of either organic or inorganic acids. Anion gap is calculated as follows:

   Anion gap = $Na^+ - (Cl^- + HCO_3^-)$.

   Normal anion gap acidosis (12 ± 2 mEg/L) is reflected in an increase in serum $Cl^-$ and a decrease in $HCO_3^-$ from loss of alkali or from renal defects.

5. **Additional laboratory studies:** Blood urea nitrogen (BUN), creatinine, serum albumin (decreased levels may affect ABG interpretation), glucose, serum osmolality, ketones, lactate salicylate level, and toxicology screen (ethanol, cocaine, crystal methamphetamine, ecstacy) may help identify the underlying cause.

6. **Electrocardiogram (ECG):** An ECG detects dysrhythmias caused by hyperkalemia. Changes seen with hyperkalemia include peaked T waves, depressed ST segment, decreased size of R waves, decrease in or absence of P waves, and widened QRS complex. Acidosis can also cause nonspecific ECG changes.

## Collaborative Management

1. **Sodium bicarbonate (NaHCO$_3$):** May be indicated when arterial pH is 7.10 or lower. The usual mode of delivery is intravenous (IV) infusion: 2 to 3 ampules (44.5 mEq/ampule) in 1000 milliliters (mL) of 5% dextrose in water (D$_5$W). Concentration depends on the severity of the acidosis and the presence of any serum sodium disorders. NaHCO$_3$ must be given cautiously to avoid metabolic alkalosis (overshoot alkalosis), hypokalemia, hypernatremia, and pulmonary edema. Serum HCO$_3^-$ and ABGs should be assessed 30 minutes after the infusion. The goal is to increase the pH to 7.20 to 7.25. Use of NaHCO$_3$ is controversial, especially when tissue hypoxia is present with lactate accumulation (i.e., shock, sepsis, cardiac arrest) because of the potential of worsening the acidosis (see point #4 for treatment of the underlying disorder).

2. **Potassium replacement:** Hyperkalemia is usually present, but a potassium deficit can occur as well. If a potassium deficit exists (potassium ion [K$^+$] < 3.5), it must be corrected before NaHCO$_3$ is administered because when the acidosis is corrected the potassium shifts back to the intracellular spaces. This could result in serum hypokalemia with serious consequences, such as cardiac irritability with fatal dysrhythmias and generalized muscle weakness (see Chapter 8 for more information).

3. **Mechanical ventilation:** If necessary, it is important that the patient's compensatory hyperventilation be allowed to continue to prevent acidosis from becoming more severe. Therefore the respiratory rate on the ventilator should not be set lower than the rate at which the patient has been breathing spontaneously, and the tidal volume should be large enough to maintain compensatory hyperventilation until the underlying disorder can be resolved.

4. **Treatment of the underlying disorder:**
   - *DKA:* Insulin and fluids. If acidosis is severe (with a pH of < 7.10 or HCO$_3^-$ of 6 to 8 mEq/L), NaHCO$_3$ may be necessary, although its use is controversial. Use of exogenous bicarbonate can cause a profound alkalosis once the body begins to convert the ketones to HCO$_3^-$ as DKA responds to treatment.

- *Alcoholism-related ketoacidosis:* Glucose and saline solution. Monitor phosphorous levels to detect/avoid refeeding syndrome. (Severe hypophosphatemia can occur 12 to 24 hours after admission.)
- *Diarrhea:* Usually occurs in association with other fluid and electrolyte disturbances; correction addresses concurrent imbalances.
- *Acute renal failure:* Hemodialysis or peritoneal dialysis to restore an adequate level of plasma bicarbonate (see Chapter 22).
- *RTA:* May require modest amounts (< 100 mEq/day) of bicarbonate.
- *Poisoning and drug toxicity:* Treatment depends on the drug ingested or infused. Hemodialysis or peritoneal dialysis may be necessary.
- *Lactic acidosis:* Correction of the underlying disorder. Mortality associated with lactic acidosis is high. Use of $NaHCO_3$ is controversial and may worsen acidosis if tissue hypoxia is present. $NaHCO_3$ may be given in small amounts to keep the pH higher than 7.10 with frequent monitoring of mixed venous pH. If excessive bicarbonate is given, an overshoot alkalosis may occur as the lactic acidosis is corrected and lactate is converted to $HCO_3^-$.

## Nursing Diagnoses and Interventions

Nursing diagnoses and interventions are specific to the pathophysiologic process. In addition, see the section in Chapter 13 on acute respiratory acidosis for the following: "Acute confusion related to disturbance in acid-base regulation," pp. 179-180; "Impaired oral mucous membrane related to abnormal breathing pattern," pp. 180-181; "Disturbed sleep pattern related to frequent treatments and procedures," p. 181; and "Ineffective family coping related to stress reaction," pp. 181-182.

## Chronic Metabolic Acidosis

Most often, chronic metabolic acidosis is seen with chronic renal failure in which the kidneys' ability to excrete acids (endogenous and exogenous) is exceeded by acid production and ingestion. The $HCO_3^-$ in patients with end-stage renal failure usually decreases to 15 to 20 mEq/L. Treatment is indicated to maintain $HCO_3^-$ concentration at 18–20 mEq/L or higher. Respiratory compensation does occur but only to a limited degree. A modest decrease in $Paco_2$ is noted on ABG values (see Box 15-1).

## Assessment

1. **Clinical manifestations:** Usually the patient is asymptomatic, although fatigue, malaise, and anorexia may be present in relation to the underlying disease
2. **History and risk factors:** Chronic renal failure and RTA

## Diagnostic Tests

1. **ABG values:** $Paco_2$ is less than 35 mm Hg; pH is less than 7.40 (in advanced renal failure, the pH is ~7.30).
2. **Total $CO_2$:** Is less than 24 mEq/L (usually 15 to 18 mEq/L). With severe acidosis, it is 12 mEq/L or lower.
3. **Serum electrolytes:** The serum calcium level is checked before treatment of acidosis is initiated to prevent tetany induced by hypocalcemia (caused by a decrease in ionized calcium). The serum potassium level should be monitored after acidosis has been corrected to detect hypokalemia because potassium shifts back into the cells.

## Collaborative Management

1. **Alkalizing agents:** To maintain $HCO_3^-$ concentration at 18 to 20 mEq/L, oral alkali are administered (e.g., $NaHCO_3$ tablets, Shol's solution). They are used cautiously to prevent fluid overload and tetany caused by hypocalcemia. Sodium citrate should be avoided because it may increase aluminum absorption. (This is a particular problem if aluminum hydroxide is used to control hyperphosphatemia.) NOTE: Be alert to the possibility of pulmonary edema if oliguria is present and bicarbonate is administered parenterally. Chronic acidosis is of concern with chronic renal failure because the bones are used as a chronic buffer and this contributes to renal bone disease. Metabolic acidosis can also lead to increased skeletal muscle breakdown, leading to weakness. Metabolic acidosis causes an increase in ammonium production that can lead to nephron injury, which speeds up the progression of kidney disease.

2. **Hemodialysis or peritoneal dialysis:** If indicated by chronic renal failure or other disease processes. Uncontrolled acidosis may be an indicator of the need for initiating or increasing dialytic therapy in patients with chronic renal failure.

3. **Dietary restrictions:** Low-protein diet decreases daily acid load improving chronic acidosis. Fluid restriction may also be indicated.

## Nursing Diagnoses and Interventions

**Imbalanced nutrition: less than body requirements** related to decreased intake from fatigue, dietary restrictions, and metallic taste in the mouth (caused by uremic state).

**Desired outcome:** The patient's weight remains stable.

1. Provide foods that correspond to the patient's prescribed diet and preferences.

2. Offer small meals and snacks at frequent intervals.

3. Offer oral care often to minimize the metallic taste. Brushing teeth before meals and using mouthwash frequently throughout the day are helpful.

4. Provide hard candy to keep the oral mucosa moist, diminish metallic taste, and supply calories.

5. Monitor hemoglobin and hematocrit levels to determine whether anemia may be contributing to the patient's fatigue.

6. Provide periods of uninterrupted rest by clustering necessary treatments and procedures. If possible, avoid performing unpleasant or uncomfortable treatments in the 1 hour before and after mealtimes.

7. Encourage family members to eat with the patient or be present at mealtimes to provide social interaction.

Other nursing diagnoses and interventions are specific to the underlying pathophysiologic process.

# Metabolic Alkalosis

16

## Acute Metabolic Alkalosis

Acute metabolic alkalosis is a disorder that results in an elevated serum bicarbonate, greater than 24 milliequivalents/liter (mEq/L), and a pH greater than 7.40 as a result of hydrogen ion ($H^+$) loss or excess alkali intake. Most causes of metabolic alkalosis can be classified in two basic groups: $Cl^-$ depletion or $K^+$ depletion with mineral-corticosteroid excess. These include loss of gastric acid (from vomiting or nasogastric [NG] suction) and diuretic use. Posthypercapneic alkalosis, which occurs when chronic carbon dioxide ($CO_2$) retention is corrected rapidly, and excessive sodium bicarbonate administration (e.g., overcorrection of metabolic acidosis) are less common causes. A compensatory increase in partial pressure of carbon dioxide in arterial blood ($Pa_{CO_2}$) up to 50 to 60 millimeters of mercury (mm Hg) is seen in patients with normal lung function. Respiratory compensation is limited because of hypoxemia, which develops from decreased alveolar ventilation. Severe metabolic alkalosis ( $> 7.55$) has a high mortality rate.

## Assessment

1. **Clinical manifestations:** Muscular weakness, neuromuscular instability, hyporeflexia, polyuria, and polydipsia occur from accompanying hypokalemia. Signs of volume depletion (e.g., postural hypotension, decreased jugular venous pressure, poor skin turgor) may also be present. Severe alkalosis can result in signs of neuromuscular excitability (e.g., tetany) and apathy, confusion, and stupor.
2. **Electrocardiogram (ECG) findings:** Numerous types of atrial-ventricular dysrhythmias as a result of the cardiac irritability that occurs with hypokalemia; changes in the T and U waves may be noted.

3. **History and risk factors (Box 16-1):**
   ■ *Clinical circumstances associated with volume/chloride ($Cl^-$) depletion:*
   Vomiting
   Bulimia

---

### Box 16-1    Causes of Metabolic Alkalosis

$Cl^-$ Depletion

■ Loss of gastric secretions*: vomiting, NG drainage, bulimia
■ $Cl^-$ wasting diuretics*: thiazides, loop diuretics
■ Diarrhea: congenital chloridorrhea, villous adenoma
■ Postchronic hypercapnia
■ Cystic fibrosis

$K^+$ Depletion (mineral-corticoid excess)

■ Primary aldosteronism: adenoma, idiopathic hyperplasia
■ Secondary aldosteronism: adrenal corticosteroid excess, severe hypertension, renal cell carcinoma
■ Apparent mineral-corticoid excess: primary deoxycorticosterone excess, licorice, carbenoxolone, Liddle's syndrome
■ Laxative abuse, clay ingestion
■ Bartter's syndrome

Hypercalcemic States

■ Hypercalcemia of malignancy
■ Acute/chronic milk alkali syndrome

Miscellaneous Causes

■ Medication: bicarbonate ingestion (massive or with renal insufficiency), carbenicillin, ampicillin, penicillin
■ Refeeding after starvation
■ Hypoproteinemia

---

Modified from Galla J: Metabolic alkalosis. In Dubose T, Hamm L, editors: *Acid-base and electrolyte disorders: a companion to Brenner & Rector's The Kidney,* Philadelphia, 2003, WB Saunders.
*Most common causes.

Gastric drainage

Thiazide diuretics

- *Aldosteronism:* Primary aldosteronism (adenoma) or secondary aldosteronism (severe hypertension, renal cell cancer) or mineral-corticoid excess (licorice consumption).
- *Posthypercapneic alkalosis:* When chronic $CO_2$ retention is rapidly corrected, the compensatory increase in serum bicarbonate ion ($HCO_3^-$) is still present and can lead to a profound alkalosis.
- *Excessive alkali intake:* May be iatrogenic from overcorrection of metabolic acidosis (frequently seen during cardiopulmonary resuscitation [CPR]). Excessive ingestion of sodium bicarbonate ($NaHCO_3$; e.g., baking soda, Alka-Seltzer) or calcium carbonate (e.g., Tums, Rolaids) is another potential cause if renal insufficiency is already present and $HCO_3^-$ excretion is affected.
- *Laxative abuse/clay ingestion.*

## Diagnostic Tests

1. **Arterial blood gas (ABG) values:** The severity of alkalosis and response to therapy should be determined. The pH is greater than 7.40. In severe metabolic alkalosis, the $Paco_2$ can exceed 60 mm Hg as a compensatory response (in the absence of underlying lung disease).
2. **Total $CO_2$:** Values are elevated to greater than 28 mEq/L.
3. **Serum electrolytes:** Usually, serum potassium ($K^+$) is low (< 4 mEq/L), as is serum $Cl^-$ (< 95 mEq/L). Although the relationship between metabolic alkalosis and $K^+$ is not completely understood, alkalosis and hypokalemia often occur together.
4. **Urine electrolytes:** It is helpful before starting therapy to differentiate between causes of metabolic alkalosis.
5. **ECG:** To assess for dysrhythmias, especially if profound alkalosis or hypokalemia is present.

## Collaborative Management

Management depends on the underlying disorder. Mild or moderate metabolic alkalosis usually does not require specific therapeutic interventions.

1. **Saline infusion:** Isotonic saline infusion may correct volume ($Cl^-$) deficit in patients with alkalosis from gastric

losses, diuretics, or posthypercapnia. Metabolic alkalosis is difficult to correct if hypovolemia and $Cl^-$ deficit are not corrected.

2. **Potassium chloride (KCl):** Indicated for patients with low $K^+$ levels. KCl is preferred over other $K^+$ salts because $Cl^-$ losses can be replaced simultaneously.

3. **Histamine $H_2$ receptor antagonists (e.g., cimetidine, ranitidine, famotidine):** Reduce production of gastric hydrochloric acid (HCl) and therefore useful in preventing or decreasing the metabolic alkalosis that can occur with gastric suctioning.

4. **Carbonic anhydrase inhibitors:** Acetazolamide (Diamox) is especially useful for correcting metabolic alkalosis for patients who cannot tolerate rapid volume expansion (e.g., individuals with congestive heart failure). It can be given orally or intravenously. Acetazolamide causes a large increase in renal secretion of $HCO_3^-$ and $K^+$; therefore it may be necessary to supplement potassium before or during administration of the medication.

5. **Acidifying agents:** Severe metabolic alkalosis (pH, $> 7.55$; and $HCO_3^-$, 40 to 45 mEq/L) may require treatment with acidifying agents such as diluted HCl, ammonium chloride ($NH_4Cl$), or arginine hydrochloride. HCl infusions must be administered through a central line; $NH_4Cl$ may be given peripherally and is contraindicated in patients with hepatic or renal insufficiency. Because of the serious side effects, these medications are not commonly used.

## Nursing Diagnoses and Interventions

Nursing diagnoses and interventions are specific to the underlying pathophysiologic process. In addition, the following may apply:

**Decreased cardiac output** related to electric factors from metabolic alkalosis induced by gastric suctioning or potassium-wasting diuretics.

**Desired outcome:** ECG reveals a normal tracing; pH is 7.45 or lower.

1. Monitor laboratory values, especially pH and serum $CO_2$, to determine the patient's response to therapy. Notify the physician if there are significant changes or a lack of response to treatment. (pH should be assessed 20 to 30 minutes after

pharmacologic intervention to assess response to treatment.)

2. Monitor the ECG for the presence of dysrhythmias. Assess apical and radial pulses simultaneously when evaluating cardiac rate and rhythm to detect pulse deficit. Notify the physician of any changes in cardiac rate and rhythm.

3. Monitor patient response to saline infusion by assessing rate and depth of respiration and lung sounds. (Patients with congestive heart failure may be sensitive to small increases in circulating volume.)

4. Monitor $K^+$ levels, especially in patients receiving digitalis preparations. (Recall that hypokalemia frequently coexists with metabolic alkalosis.) Consult with the physician if $K^+$ levels drop below 3.5 mEq/L. Hypokalemia sensitizes patients to the cardiotoxic effect of digitalis. When KCl infusion is ordered, assess site of peripheral infusion frequently looking for signs of extravasation. KCl is irritating to tissue; if extravasation and irritation occur, stop infusion immediately, remove the intravenous catheter, notify the physician, and apply compresses, warm or cold depending on the irritant.

5. Use isotonic saline solutions to irrigate gastric tubes. Water is not recommended for irrigation because it can cause a washout of electrolytes.

6. If the patient is permitted to have ice chips, administer limited quantities to avoid washing electrolytes from the patient's stomach. The total volume of ice consumed over a shift is frequently underestimated. Determine the volume of a specific number of ice cubes or the quantity of crushed ice by melting and measuring. Establish the volume of fluid the patient may consume each shift. Document the volume consumed in milliliters (mL) or ounces (oz), not by the number of cubes.

7. Measure and document the amount of fluid removed with suction.

8. Weigh the patient daily to determine fluid volume status.

9. Administer a histamine $H_2$ receptor antagonist (e.g., cimetidine, ranitidine, famotidine) as prescribed to block hydrochloride secretion by the stomach, thus lessening systemic metabolic alkalosis in patients undergoing NG suctioning.

# Chronic Metabolic Alkalosis

Chronic metabolic alkalosis results in a pH greater than 7.40. $Pa_{CO_2}$ is elevated ($>45$ mm Hg) to compensate for the loss of $H^+$ or excess serum $HCO_3^-$. There are three clinical situations in which this can occur: 1, abnormalities in the kidneys' excretion of $HCO_3^-$ related to a mineral-corticoid effect; 2, loss of $H^+$ through the gastrointestinal (GI) tract; and 3, diuretic therapy.

## Assessment

1. **Clinical manifestations:** The patient may be asymptomatic. With severe $K^+$ depletion and profound alkalosis, the patient may experience weakness, neuromuscular instability, and a decrease in GI tract motility, which can result in an ileus with an absence of bowel sounds.
2. **ECG findings:** Frequent premature ventricular contractions or U waves with hypokalemia and alkalosis.
3. **History and risk factors:**
   - *Diuretic use:* Thiazide diuretics cause a loss of $Cl^-$, $K^+$, and $H^+$. Massive depletion of $K^+$ stores with a loss of up to 1000 mEq (which is one third of the total body $K^+$) may occur, causing profound hypokalemia ($K^+ < 2$ mEq).
   - *Hyperadrenocorticism:* Cushing's syndrome and primary aldosteronism cause a mild to moderate alkalosis. More severe hypokalemic alkalosis is seen with adrenocorticotropic hormone (ACTH)–secreting tumors (primarily tumors of the lungs). Increased production of ACTH at the ectopic site leads to an increase in $H^+$ secretion and a chronic loss of $K^+$, which leads to total body depletion of $K^+$ with profound hypokalemia ($K^+ < 2$ mEq/L).
   - *Chronic vomiting or chronic GI losses through gastric suction*
   - *Milk alkali syndrome:* An infrequent cause of metabolic alkalosis. Hypercalcemic nephropathy and alkalosis develop from excessive intake of absorbable alkali.
   - *Cystic fibrosis:* Large amounts of $Cl^-$ can be lost through sweat.

## Diagnostic Tests

1. **ABG values:** Determine the severity of acid-base imbalance. $Pa_{CO_2}$ is increased ($>45$ mm Hg), and the pH is greater than 7.4.

2. **Total CO$_2$:** Is greater than 28 mEq/L.
3. **Serum electrolytes:** Usually K$^+$ is profoundly low (may be < 2 mEq/L). Cl$^-$ may be less than 95 mEq/L, and magnesium may be less than 1.5 mEq/L. Hypomagnesemia may contribute to irritability of the myocardium.

## Collaborative Management

The goal is to correct the underlying acid-base disorder via the following interventions:

1. **Fluid management:** If volume depletion exists, isotonic saline infusions are given.
2. **Potassium replacement:** If a Cl$^-$ deficit is also present, KCl is the drug of choice. If a Cl$^-$ deficit does not exist, other K$^+$ salts are acceptable.
   - *Intravenous potassium:* If the patient is on a cardiac monitor, up to 20 mEq/hour of KCl is given for serious hypokalemia. Concentrated doses of KCl (> 40 mEq/L) require administration through a central venous line because of blood vessel irritation.
   - *Oral potassium:* This tastes unpleasant. Most patients can tolerate only 15 mEq per glass, with a maximum daily dose of 60 to 80 mEq. Slow-release potassium tablets are an acceptable form of KCl. All forms of KCl may be irritating to gastric or intestinal mucosa.
   - *Dietary:* A normal diet contains 3 g, or 75 mEq, of K$^+$ but not in the form of KCl. Dietary supplementation of K$^+$ is not effective if a concurrent Cl$^-$ deficit is also present.
3. **Potassium-sparing diuretics:** May be added to the treatment plan if thiazide diuretics are the cause of hypokalemia and metabolic alkalosis.
4. **Identification and correction of the cause of hyperadrenocorticism.**

## Nursing Diagnoses and Interventions

**Deficient knowledge** related to necessary precautions for taking thiazide diuretics.
**Desired outcome:** The patient verbalizes knowledge about thiazide diuretics and necessary precautions that must be taken.

1. Provide the patient and significant others with the following information about the prescribed thiazide diuretic: name, purpose, dosage, precautions, and potential side effects.

2. Stress the importance of taking only the prescribed dose; higher concentrations of the medication increase the risk of hypokalemia and alkalosis.
3. Explain that diets high in sodium increase the risk of alkalosis and hypokalemia, necessitating restrictions of sodium as prescribed.
4. If KCl supplements are prescribed, teach the patient the following:
   - Oral potassium has an unpleasant taste and is most palatable when mixed with orange juice or tomato juice.
   - Slow-release tablets should not be chewed.
   - Oral potassium and slow-release potassium tablets can irritate the stomach and should be taken with meals.
   - Although many foods contain potassium, they should not be used as a substitute for the KCl supplements prescribed by the patient's physician.

For other nursing diagnoses and interventions, see the section on acute metabolic alkalosis for the following: "Decreased cardiac output related to electric factors (risk of dysrhythmias) from metabolic alkalosis induced by gastric suctioning or potassium-wasting diuretics," pp. 204-205.

# Mixed Acid-Base Disorders

17

A mixed acid-base disturbance occurs when two or more simple acid-base disorders are present at the same time. The effect of a mixed acid-base disturbance on pH depends on both the specific disorders involved and their severity. If a mixed disorder involves two types of acidosis, a larger drop in pH can be expected than would occur if a mixed acidosis-alkalosis disorder were present. When two opposing disorders (i.e., an acidosis and an alkalosis) occur simultaneously, the pH is determined by the predominant disorder. In some cases, the pH is normal in the presence of a mixed acid-base disorder (Table 17-1).

## Case Study One

A 19-year-old woman with a history of type 1 diabetes mellitus (DM) is seen with a 2-day history of nausea, vomiting, polyuria, and polydipsia. She is febrile and has orthostatic hypotension (blood pressure [BP], 117/78 millimeters of mercury [mm Hg] supine and 92/60 mm Hg sitting with feet over the side of the bed). The patient is in respiratory distress indicated by use of accessory muscles; rales and wheezing are present bilaterally on physical examination.

## Values

| pH | $Pa_{CO_2}$ | $Pa_{O_2}$ | $HCO_3^-$ | $Na^+$ | $K^+$ | $Cl^-$ | Glucose | Anion Gap |
|------|------|------|------|------|------|------|------|------|
| 7.15 | 45 mm Hg | 68 mm Hg | 15 mEq/L | 123 | 4.5 | 80 | 357 | 28 |

Anion gap determination: $123 - (80 + 15) = 28$ $\quad Na^+ \quad Cl^- \quad HCO_3^-$

Table 17-1    Mixed acid-base disorders

| Types | Examples |
|---|---|
| Metabolic acidosis and metabolic acidosis | Renal failure, diarrhea |
| Acute respiratory acidosis and chronic respiratory acidosis | Pneumonia, emphysema |
| Metabolic acidosis and metabolic alkalosis | Diabetic ketoacidosis, vomiting |
| Metabolic acidosis and respiratory acidosis | Lactic acidosis, respiratory arrest |
| Metabolic acidosis and respiratory alkalosis | Ethylene glycol ingestion, pneumonia |
| Metabolic alkalosis and respiratory acidosis | Gastric suction, sedative overdose |
| Metabolic alkalosis and respiratory alkalosis | Diuretic use, hepatic failure |

## Analysis

Step 1: pH is abnormal, indicates a severe acidosis.

Step 2: $Paco_2$ is at the upper limit of normal, moving toward acidosis (moving in the opposite direction as the pH).

Step 3: $HCO_3^-$ is decreased and moving in the same direction as the pH, indicating metabolic acidosis.

Step 4: The $HCO_3^-$ is significantly decreased; the $Paco_2$ is in the normal range, but the expected $Paco_2$ should be 29. (The $Paco_2$ should decrease 1.2 mm Hg for every 1 mEq/L decrease in $HCO_3^-$). See Table 12-4. The "elevated" $Paco_2$ indicates the presence of respiratory acidosis.

Step 5: Anion gap assessment shows a high anion gap metabolic acidosis. (History and symptoms point to diabetic ketoacidosis as the cause.)

## Evaluation

The patient has a complex mixed acid-base disorder: metabolic acidosis and respiratory acidosis. The respiratory dysfunction has led to a more severe acidosis because normal respiratory compensation is not available. (In a healthy young patient, the maximum respiratory compensation decreases $Paco_2$ to 10 to 15 mm Hg; in a healthy older adult, a decreased $Paco_2$ to 20 mm Hg is normal.) A rising $Paco_2$ in the face of metabolic acidosis is cause for concern because any further worsening of pulmonary function and subsequent rise in $Paco_2$ can lead to an abrupt decrease in pH.

## Case Study Two

The patient is a 67-year-old man. He is seen with a 4-day history of shortness of breath; his history includes congestive heart failure, smoking, and recent change in diuretic and dose. Physical findings include adventitious breath sounds bilaterally, peripheral edema, and a wet cough. The patient is alert and oriented.

## Values

| pH | $Paco_2$ | $HCO_3^-$ | $Na^+$ | $Cl^-$ | $K^+$ | Anion Gap |
|---|---|---|---|---|---|---|
| 7.45 | 65 mm Hg | 44 mEq/L | 144 | 86 | 3.0 | 14 |

$$Na^+ \quad Cl^- \quad HCO_3^-$$
Anion gap determination: $144 - (86 + 3\ 44) = 14$

## Analysis

Step 1: pH is normal, leaning toward alkalosis.

Step 2: $Paco_2$ is high. Chronic respiratory acidosis is present, although the pH does not reflect the degree of respiratory dysfunction from renal compensation.

Step 3: $HCO_3^-$ is high. A renal compensatory response raises the $HCO_3^-$ 3.5 mEq/L for every 10 mm Hg increase in $Paco_2$, leading to an anticipated $HCO_3^-$ of 31 mEq/L. The current level exceeds the amount by 13 mEq/L. In addition to renal compensation, an acute coexisting metabolic alkalosis is present. The patient has a history of recent diuretic use and a serum $Cl^-$ of 86, supporting the assessment of metabolic alkalosis.

Step 4: Anion gap is normal.

## Evaluation

Patient has a mixed acid-base disturbance: chronic respiratory acidosis and metabolic alkalosis. A normal pH in the face of an increased $HCO_3^-$ and an elevated $Paco_2$ suggests a mixed disorder, not a compensatory response. The disorders balance or cancel each other, leading to a normal pH. Compensation cannot return a pH to normal except in cases of chronic respiratory alkalosis.

The patient is alert and oriented, with a high $Paco_2$. This lends support to the assessment of a chronic respiratory acidosis. A patient with an acute increase in $Paco_2$ to 65 mm Hg would present with restlessness, asterixis, and other neurologic and physical manifestations. The chronic nature of the respiratory imbalance also supports the assessment of a chronic compensatory alkalosis with a super imposed metabolic alkalosis from recent diuretic use. (The compensatory renal response takes 3 to 5 days to reach maximum compensation, further supporting the evidence of a chronic respiratory disorder.)

## Case Study Three

A 48-year-old woman is seen with nausea, vomiting, and severe abdominal pain. A bowel obstruction is diagnosed.

### Values

| pH | $Paco_2$ | $HCO_3^-$ | $Na^+$ | $Cl^-$ | $K^+$ | Anion Gap |
|------|----------|-----------|--------|--------|-------|-----------|
| 7.33 | 35 mm Hg | 18 mEq/L | 145 | 85 | 4.0 | 32 |

$$Na^+ \quad Cl^- \quad HCO_3^-$$
Anion gap determination: $145 - (85 + 18) = 32$

### Analysis

Step 1: pH is decreased, indicating an acidosis.
Step 2: $Paco_2$ is in the normal range.
Step 3: $HCO_3^-$ is low and moving in the same direction as the pH.
Step 4: Anion gap is 32, indicating a high anion gap acidosis. The cause of the acidosis is the accumulation of

lactic acid from the ischemic bowel. With this large of an anion gap, the $HCO_3^-$ would be expected to be lower, indicating a coexisting metabolic alkalosis. (NOTE: See the decreased $Cl^-$ value.)

## Evaluation

At first glance, the patient appears to have a mild lactic acidosis. On further evaluation, a metabolic alkalosis is discovered masking the severity of the acidosis. The root cause of the metabolic alkalosis is vomiting and subsequent nasogastric suctioning. The patient is experiencing a severe metabolic acidosis and a coexisting metabolic alkalosis.

## Case Study Four

The patient is a 73-year-old man admitted with a history of cirrhosis and prolonged diarrhea (of 3 days' duration). He is alert and oriented but has muscle weakness.

## Values

| pH | $Pa_{CO_2}$ | $HCO_3^-$ | $Na^+$ | $K^+$ | $Cl^-$ | Anion Gap |
|----|-------------|-----------|--------|-------|--------|-----------|
| 7.38 | 28 mm Hg | 13 mEq/L | 138 | 2.9 | 115 | 10 |

$$Na^+ \quad Cl^- \quad HCO_3^-$$
Anion gap determination: $138 - (115 + 13) = 10$

## Analysis

Step 1: pH is normal.
Step 2: $Pa_{CO_2}$ is low; respiratory alkalosis is present.
Step 3: $HCO_3^-$ is low; metabolic acidosis is present. With this degree of metabolic acidosis, the pH is expected to be lower.
Step 4: Anion gap is normal.

## Evaluation

Cirrhosis stimulates the respiratory center, resulting in respiratory alkalosis. Prolonged diarrhea has resulted in the loss of $HCO_3^-$, leading to metabolic acidosis with a normal anion gap. Over time, respiratory alkalosis can result in a compensatory decrease in serum $HCO_3^-$, but normally serum $HCO_3^-$ does not decrease to less than 16 mEq/L as a compensatory measure. Therefore these values, along with the patient's history, reflect a mixed acid-base disorder: respiratory alkalosis and metabolic acidosis. The pH is in the normal range because the opposing disorders, respiratory alkalosis and metabolic acidosis, have "balanced" each other. (The symptom of muscle weakness is related to the hypokalemia.)

# CLINICAL CONDITIONS ASSOCIATED WITH FLUID, ELECTROLYTE, AND ACID-BASE IMBALANCE

**III**

# Gastrointestinal Disorders 18

The gastrointestinal (GI) tract plays an important role in maintaining fluid and electrolyte balance because, in health, it is the primary site of fluid and electrolyte gain (see Chapter 3). Approximately 1.5 to 2 liters (L) of fluid are gained each day through the consumption of fluids and solid food. In addition, approximately 6 L of fluid are secreted into and reabsorbed from the GI tract daily, equaling approximately half of the extracellular fluid (ECF) volume. Despite this large volume, the GI tract only minimally contributes to normal fluid loss (approximately 100 to 200 milliliters [mL]/day). In disease, however, the GI tract becomes the most common site of abnormal fluid and electrolyte loss, potentially resulting in profound acid-base and fluid and electrolyte imbalance.

The composition of the GI secretions varies with the location within the GI tract (Table 18-1). Therefore the nature of the fluid and electrolyte imbalance varies with the type of fluid lost. GI fluids include saliva and bile and gastric, pancreatic, and intestinal secretions. GI disorders causing fluid and electrolyte loss may be differentiated into the loss of upper GI contents and the loss of lower GI contents.

## Loss Of Upper Gastrointestinal Contents

Upper GI secretions include saliva and gastric juices. Losses may occur because of problems such as vomiting and procedures such as gastric suction. (Box 18-1 lists potential causes of vomiting.)

### Saliva

Approximately 1 L of saliva is produced each day. Saliva begins the digestive process by initiating the breakdown of starches. In addition, it lubricates food, facilitating swallowing. Food and

Table 18-1   Volume and composition of GI secretions*

| Secretion | L/24 hours | Na$^+$ (mEq/L) | K$^+$ (mEq/L) | Cl$^-$ (mEq/L) | HCO$_3^-$ (mEq/L) |
|---|---|---|---|---|---|
| Saliva | 1 | 40 | 15 | 30 | 0 |
| Gastric juice | 1–2 | 40 | 7 | 100 | 0 |
| Pancreatic juice | 1–2 | 130 | 7 | 60 | 100 |
| Bile | 1 | 150 | 7 | 80 | 30 |
| Intestinal secretions | 1–2 | 140 | 5 | Variable | Variable |

*Values are approximate.

## Box 18-1   Potential Causes of Vomiting

- GI infection
- Inner ear infection
- Certain medications (e.g., chemotherapy)
- Pregnancy
- Small bowel obstruction
- Pyloric stenosis
- Uremia
- Binge-purge syndrome
- Pancreatitis
- Hepatitis
- Diabetic ketoacidosis (DKA)

saliva move through the esophagus to the stomach by peristalsis (rhythmic contractions). Once in the stomach, food and saliva are exposed to acidic secretions (see the subsequent "Gastric Juices"). Abnormal loss of saliva may occur in individuals who are unable to swallow oral secretions (e.g., those who are comatose).

### Gastric Juices

Approximately 1 to 2 L of gastric juices are produced daily; they contain hydrochloric acid, which aids digestion by breaking down food; the enzyme pepsin, which initiates digestion of proteins; and intrinsic factor, which facilitates the absorption of vitamin B$_{12}$ in the ileum.

Only alcohol and a limited amount of water are absorbed from the stomach. Most of the stomach contents move by peristalsis into the small intestine. Although the fluid and electrolyte content of food is variable, gastric contents mix and become similar in concentration to the ECF because of osmotic shifts of water into and out of the stomach. Losses from the upper GI tract (above the pylorus) are essentially isotonic and contain sodium ($Na^+$), potassium ($K^+$), chloride ($Cl^-$), and hydrogen ($H^+$; see Table 18-1).

## Gastric Suction

Gastric suction, whether via a nasogastric (NG) or orogastric (OG) tube, is a common medical procedure used to decompress the stomach. Removal of gastric contents may lead to multiple fluid and electrolyte imbalances and requires adequate parenteral replacement. This may be accomplished by administering an intravenous (IV) solution developed specifically for gastric fluid replacement (e.g., Isolyte G, made by McGaw) or customizing a solution to meet an individual patient's needs, on the basis of serum electrolyte levels. Important nursing considerations for minimizing electrolyte imbalance with gastric suction include the following:

- **Give the patient nothing by mouth** (NPO status).
- **Avoid giving ice by mouth or irrigating the catheter with plain water** because these actions increase the loss of electrolytes because of "washout." If patients are allowed ice chips, give small amounts (<1 ounce [oz]) hourly.
- **Provide frequent oral care** to minimize thirst and maximize comfort.
- **Irrigate the gastric tube with isotonic sodium chloride (NaCl) solution only.** If the catheter is irrigated and an equal amount is not withdrawn and discarded, the extra irrigant should be added to the intake record to avoid overestimation of the fluid loss.

## Potential Fluid, Electrolyte, and Acid-Base Disturbances with Loss of Upper Gastrointestinal Contents

1. **Hypovolemia:** Caused by abnormal fluid loss (see Chapter 6).
2. **Hyponatremia:** Caused by loss of $Na^+$-rich fluids with inadequate electrolyte replacement or caused by antidiuretic

hormone (ADH) and thirst-induced retention of water (see Chapter 7).

3. **Hypokalemia:** Caused by loss of $K^+$-containing fluids with inadequate replacement. Increased production of aldosterone from hypovolemia contributes to the development of hypokalemia caused by increased renal losses. NOTE: Aldosterone causes both increased retention of $Na^+$ and increased excretion of $K^+$ (see Chapter 8).

4. **Hypomagnesemia:** Caused by prolonged loss of upper GI fluids with inadequate replacement (see Chapter 11).

5. **Metabolic alkalosis:** Caused by the loss of fluids rich in $Cl^-$ and $H^+$. Hypovolemia contributes to the development and perpetuation of metabolic alkalosis as a result of volume-induced conservation of sodium bicarbonate ($NaHCO_3$; see Chapter 16).

## Loss of Lower Gastrointestinal Contents

The small intestines are the primary site of nutrient, electrolyte, and water absorption. Approximately 6 L of fluid enter the small intestines from the upper GI tract daily, of which 75% is absorbed (and returned to the ECF). The colon receives only 1 to 2 L of fluid from the ileum; all of this is usually absorbed, except 100 to 200 mL of water and a small quantity of electrolytes. Lower GI secretions include pancreatic juice, bile, and intestinal secretions.

Losses from the lower GI tract (below the pylorus) are generally isotonic and contain $Na^+$, $K^+$, and bicarbonate. Lower GI contents may be lost through diarrhea, intestinal fistulas, or intestinal resection. Diarrhea is the most common cause of lower GI fluid loss, especially in children. In developed countries, diarrhea accounts for a significant percentage of pediatric hospital admissions and clinic visits. In underdeveloped nations, diarrhea is a major cause of infant deaths. Abnormal losses from the small intestines of as much as 2000 mL/day may occur with the creation of a new ileostomy or with short bowel syndrome. Although the loss of water and electrolytes remains greater than with normal stool, over time ileostomy output decreases to only 300 to 500 mL/day. Fistulas (abnormal passages from the bowel to the skin) also may result in the loss of several liters of intestinal fluid daily. Vomiting

---

### Box 18-2    Potential Causes of Diarrhea

**Osmotic Diarrhea**
- Certain medications (e.g., lactulose, sorbitol)
- Malabsorption or maldigestion syndromes

**Secretory Diarrhea**
- Gastrointestinal infection
- Inflammatory bowel disease
- Emotional stress
- Pancreatic insufficiency
- Intestinal obstruction
- Abuse of laxatives (e.g., bisacodyl, castor oil)
- Carcinoma

---

can contribute to lower GI fluid loss because both gastric and duodenal contents may be lost. Losses from both the upper and lower GI tract can also occur with bowel obstruction. Acid-base balance is usually maintained when both gastric and duodenal fluids are lost because a loss of both $H^+$ (acid) and bicarbonate (base) occurs (see Box 18-2 for potential causes of diarrhea).

## Pancreatic Juice

Approximately 1 to 2 L of pancreatic juice are secreted each day. Pancreatic juice is high in bicarbonate, which neutralizes the acidic gastric contents as they enter the duodenum. It also contains enzymes that aid in the digestion of protein (trypsin), starches (amylase), and fats (lipase).

## Bile

Bile is produced by the liver and stored in the gallbladder. Water and electrolytes are continuously reabsorbed by the gallbladder mucosa so that the bile released into the duodenum may be 5 to 10 times more concentrated than the bile produced by the liver. The liver produces approximately 1 L of bile per day. Bile provides a means of excreting bilirubin (a breakdown product of hemoglobin) and aids in the digestion of fats via emulsification by bile salts. In addition to bilirubin and bile salts, bile contains water, $Na^+$, $K^+$, calcium, bicarbonate, cholesterol, and lecithin.

## Intestinal Secretions

In addition to bile and pancreatic juice, the intestines contain secretions produced by the intestinal glands. These glands secrete mucus (which helps protect the intestinal mucosa), hormones (e.g., secretin), electrolytes, and digestive enzymes. Approximately 1 to 2 L of intestinal gland secretions are produced each day. The secretion of isotonic intestinal fluids may increase dramatically with certain diseases such as cholera and other intestinal infections, after administration of certain medications such as laxatives, and with bowel obstruction (see "Bowel Obstruction," facing page).

## Diarrhea

*Diarrhea* is defined as an increased loss of fluid and electrolytes via the stool. The causes of diarrhea are divided into two main categories: 1, those causing osmotic diarrhea; and 2, those causing secretory diarrhea. Osmotic diarrhea occurs when poorly absorbable solutes are present in the colon. The unabsorbed solutes create an osmotic gradient for water to move from the ECF into the lumen of the bowel. In addition, water that normally would be reabsorbed from the bowel remains in the lumen. This is the means by which sorbitol and lactulose induce diarrhea. Malabsorption or maldigestion of carbohydrates also results in osmotic diarrhea because bacteria in the colon convert unabsorbed carbohydrates to organic acids. These organic acids create an osmotic gradient favoring the production of liquid stools. Osmotic diarrhea usually stops within 24 to 48 hours of fasting.

Water and electrolytes are both secreted into and reabsorbed from the lumen of the bowel. In normal conditions, there is net resorption, minimizing the volume of the stool. Secretory diarrhea develops when there is either increased secretion or decreased resorption of water and electrolytes. Unlike osmotic diarrhea, secretory diarrhea does not cease with fasting and is characterized by large losses of water and electrolytes. Bacterial infections cause secretory diarrhea by irritating the bowel mucosa and causing increased secretion of water and electrolytes. The diarrhea that occurs with inflammatory bowel diseases (e.g., ulcerative colitis, Crohn's disease) is believed to be the result of inflammation of the bowel wall, which causes both an increase in secretion and a decrease in resorption. The individual with inflammatory bowel disease may pass more than five stools a day, causing both physical and emotional debilitation.

## Bowel Obstruction

The type and extent of fluid and electrolyte imbalance that occurs with bowel obstruction depends on the location of the obstruction and its duration. The longer the bowel is obstructed, the more profound the fluid and electrolyte imbalance is. Lower GI loss occurs because of sequestering of fluid in the distended bowel. Several liters of fluid may collect in the intestinal lumen, leading to a dramatic increase in lumen pressure and eventual damage to the intestinal mucosa. Peritonitis may then occur if bacteria enter the peritoneal cavity through the damaged intestinal wall. The fluid sequestered in the bowel is inaccessible to the ECF, creating a separate third space. Peritonitis also causes a shift of fluid into a temporarily inaccessible third space. Normally the peritoneum aids in the rapid transport of fluid from the peritoneal cavity to the circulation. When the peritoneum becomes damaged or inflamed, fluid and electrolytes collect in the peritoneal cavity. The loss of ECF into an inaccessible third space causes a reduction in effective circulating volume, which stimulates both thirst and release of ADH, with the retention of water. These two factors lead to the eventual development of dilutional hyponatremia. Upper GI loss can occur with bowel obstruction because of the increased stimulus to vomit.

## Potential Fluid, Electrolyte, and Acid-Base Disturbances with Loss of Lower Gastrointestinal Contents

1. **Hypovolemia:** Caused by abnormal fluid loss (see Chapter 6).
2. **Hyponatremia:** Caused by loss of $Na^+$-containing fluids with inadequate electrolyte replacement or by thirst and ADH-induced retention of water (see Chapter 7).

3. **Hypokalemia:** Caused by loss of $K^+$-containing fluids, combined with inadequate replacement. Hypovolemia-induced secondary hyperaldosteronism causes increased renal loss of $K^+$ (see Chapter 8).
4. **Hypomagnesemia:** Caused by abnormal fluid loss (see Chapter 11). Typically hypomagnesemia occurs only with prolonged loss of GI fluids, as with ulcerative colitis.
5. **Metabolic acidosis:** Caused by a loss of fluids rich in bicarbonate (see Chapter 15).

# Surgical Disturbances 19

Disturbances in fluid and electrolyte balance are common in surgical patients because of a combination of preoperative, perioperative, and postoperative factors.

## Preoperative Factors

1. **Preexisting conditions** such as diabetes mellitus (DM), liver disease, or renal insufficiency may be aggravated by the stress of surgery (see Chapters 20, 22, and 24).
2. **Diagnostic procedures** such as arteriogram or intravenous pyelogram that require the administration of intravenous dyes, which may cause inappropriate urinary excretion of water and electrolytes because of the osmotic diuresis effect.
3. **Administration of medications** such as steroids or diuretics, which may affect the excretion of water and electrolytes.
4. **Surgical preparations** such as enemas or laxatives, which may act to increase fluid loss from the gastrointestinal (GI) tract (see Chapter 18).
5. **Medical management of preexisting conditions** (e.g., gastric suction, gastric lavage).
6. **Preoperative fluid restriction** (e.g., nothing by mouth [NPO status] after midnight). During an average 6-hour period of fluid restriction, a healthy adult patient loses approximately 300 to 500 milliliters (mL) of fluid through normal means. Fluid loss may be increased greatly if the patient has abnormal fluid loss or fever. Because infants and toddlers have a greater relative body surface area and a higher metabolic rate than adults, NPO status places them at increased risk for fluid loss. It is recommended that infants and toddlers be scheduled as the first surgical cases of the day.

7. **Preexisting fluid deficit,** which should be corrected before surgery to minimize the effects of anesthesia.

## Perioperative Factors

1. **Induction of anesthesia,** which may lead to the development of hypotension in patients with preoperative hypovolemia because of the loss of compensatory mechanisms such as tachycardia or vasoconstriction.
2. **Abnormal blood loss** related to preoperative trauma or to the surgical procedure itself.
3. **Abnormal loss of extracellular fluid (ECF) into a third space** (e.g., loss of ECF into the wall and lumen of the bowel during bowel surgery). This fluid is temporarily unavailable either to the intracellular fluid (ICF) or ECF; it is termed *third-space fluid.* Replacement of third-space fluid is necessary to maintain perfusion of tissues. Loss of ECF also occurs when intravascular volume is lost into a nonequilibrating space (e.g., through bleeding into a fractured hip). Fluid management during this time is the most important aspect in the hemodynamic function of a surgical patient.
4. **Evaporative loss of fluid from the surgical wound,** usually of concern with large wounds and prolonged operative procedures.
   NOTE: All of the previous factors relate to fluid volume (see Chapter 6).

## Postoperative Factors

1. **Stress** of surgery and postoperative pain, which leads to an increased release of antidiuretic hormone (ADH) by the posterior pituitary gland and of adrenocorticotropic hormone (ACTH) by the anterior pituitary gland. Increased ADH results in the retention of water by the kidneys. Excessive production may lead to the development of hyponatremia (see Chapter 7). ACTH acts on the adrenal cortex to cause an increase in the release of aldosterone and hydrocortisone. Both aldosterone and hydrocortisone lead to an increased retention of sodium and water and an increased excretion of potassium by the kidneys.

The combined effects of these hormones may result in postoperative fluid retention lasting up to 48 to 72 hours (see Chapter 6).

2. **Increase in tissue catabolism** (breakdown) from tissue trauma, which causes the patient to produce a greater than normal amount of water from oxidation (see Chapter 6).

3. **Reduction in effective circulating volume,** which stimulates production of ADH and aldosterone. Potential causes include bleeding, fluid loss from the surgical wound, abnormal sequestration of fluid (i.e., third-space shift), draining fistulas, gastric suction, vomiting, and increased insensible fluid loss from fever (see Chapter 6).

4. **Risk or presence of postoperative ileus,** which may restrict a patient's ability to take oral fluids and may necessitate gastric suction (see Chapter 18).

## Potential Fluid, Electrolyte, and Acid-Base Disturbances

1. **Hyperkalemia:** May occur during the immediate postoperative period because of the release of intracellular potassium as a result of tissue trauma (see Chapter 8). In patients with renal failure, significant hyperkalemia may occur.

2. **Metabolic acidosis:** May occur because of an abnormal production of lactic acid in a hypotensive patient with tissue hypoxia (see Chapter 15).

3. **Metabolic alkalosis:** May occur because of prolonged gastric suctioning.

4. **Respiratory acidosis:** May develop as the result of inadequate ventilation as a result of respiratory depression from anesthesia or pain medication, splinting of the operative site, or restriction to bed, increasing the risk of atelectasis or pneumonia, especially in a patient with chronic obstructive pulmonary disease (COPD) (see Chapter 13).

5. **Respiratory alkalosis:** May develop initially if hypoxemia occurs as a result of postoperative pulmonary disturbance (e.g., pneumonia, pulmonary edema, pulmonary emboli) or from anxiety from pain (see Chapter 14).

# Endocrinologic Disorders

**20**

## Diabetic Ketoacidosis

Diabetic ketoacidosis (DKA) is a life-threatening complication of diabetes mellitus (DM) that is characterized by hyperglycemia, dehydration, electrolyte imbalance, ketosis, and acidosis. The condition occurs most commonly in persons with type 1 DM who experience illness, infection, trauma, omission or inadequate use of insulin, or surgery. A relative or absolute insulin deficiency prevents the normal use of serum glucose and results in cellular starvation despite the abundance of glucose in the serum. The unmet energy requirements of the cells stimulate gluconeogenesis and glycogen conversion in the liver and trigger the release of catabolic stress hormones, which act to elevate the serum glucose even further. The body is forced to break down its fat and protein stores to meet the energy requirements of cell metabolism. The rate of breakdown exceeds the body's ability to use these alternate energy sources, however, and ketone bodies accumulate in the blood. Ketones cause the blood pH level to drop, which results in the potential for profound metabolic acidosis (positive anion gap metabolic acidosis). Hyperglycemia results in increased serum osmolality.

Glucose and ketones not reabsorbed by the renal tubule cause an osmotic diuresis, with losses of sodium, potassium, phosphorus, magnesium, and body water, which can lead to severe dehydration and hypovolemic shock. Despite significant loss of potassium in the urine, a patient may initially have normal or elevated plasma potassium because of the dramatic shift of potassium from the cells as a result of insulin deficiency, acidosis, and tissue catabolism. Increased blood viscosity and platelet aggregation can result in thromboembolism. Dehydration also decreases tissue perfusion, and the resulting lactic acid waste products exacerbate the existing metabolic acidosis. The lowered pH level stimulates the respiratory center, producing the deep rapid respirations known as *Kussmaul's* respirations. The large amount of ketones lends a fruity or acetone odor to the breath. If the condition is not treated promptly, elevated serum osmolality, acidosis, and dehydration depress consciousness to the point of coma. Death can result from hypovolemia or profound central nervous system (CNS) depression.

## Potential Fluid, Electrolyte, and Acid-Base Disturbances

1. **Fluid volume deficit** caused by polyuria from hyperglycemia and ketonemia. Initially, hypovolemia is treated with isotonic saline solution (0.9% sodium chloride [NaCl]) administered at a rapid rate. Subsequent volume replacement is with 0.45% NaCl solution, which more closely approximates the fluid loss. Once the blood glucose level falls to 250 to 300 milligrams/deciliter (mg/dL), dextrose-containing solutions are used (e.g., 5% dextrose in 0.45% NaCl or 5% dextrose in 0.225% NaCl).
2. **Hyponatremia** (initially) caused by the osmotic shift of water from the cells (pseudohyponatremia) and also by the loss of sodium in the urine (see Chapter 7).
3. **Hypernatremia** (as the disease progresses) caused by dehydration as a result of osmotic diuresis with the loss of free water (i.e., water is lost in excess of electrolytes). Hypernatremia is corrected with administration of hypotonic intravenous (IV) fluids (see Chapter 7).
4. **Hyperkalemia** (initially) caused by the movement of potassium from the cell as the result of tissue catabolism, acidosis, and insulin deficiency (see Chapter 8).
5. **Hypokalemia** (after treatment) caused by the loss of potassium as the result of osmotic diuresis and the movement of potassium back into the cell, occurring with the administration of insulin and correction of acidosis. Potassium levels may drop precipitously with treatment of DKA, necessitating frequent monitoring and aggressive potassium replacement (see Chapter 8).
6. **Hyperphosphatemia** (initially) caused by the movement of phosphorus from the cell as the result of tissue catabolism (see Chapter 10).

7. **Hypophosphatemia and hypomagnesemia** (after treatment) caused by the loss of these electrolytes as the result of osmotic diuresis and repair of the tissue with treatment. Hypophosphatemia may be corrected with replacing a portion of the potassium deficit with potassium phosphate (see Chapters 10 and 11).

8. **Metabolic acidosis** occurring with the abnormal production of ketoacids and lactic acid resulting in an increased anion gap with a pH less than 7.30 and a bicarbonate ($HCO_3^-$) less than 15. Metabolic acidosis usually reverses with the administration of insulin and fluids. Severe acidosis (pH < 7.00 to 7.10), however, may necessitate treatment with IV sodium bicarbonate ($NaHCO_3$), although this treatment is controversial (see Chapter 15).

9. **Hypochloremia** may be present initially because of the loss of chloride in the urine and the movement of water from the cells. Hyperchloremia may occur with treatment because of administration of isotonic NaCl solution, which contains chloride in a concentration that exceeds the plasma chloride level.

## Hyperosmolar Hyperglycemic Nonketotic Syndrome

Hyperosmolar hyperglycemic nonketotic (HHNK) syndrome is a life-threatening emergency characterized by severe hyperglycemia (i.e., blood glucose levels exceed 600 mg/dL and may be as high as 2000 mg/dL) with the absence of significant ketonemia. As with DKA, hyperglycemia causes an osmotic diuresis with the loss of electrolytes, including sodium, chloride, potassium, magnesium, and phosphorus. The diuresis is hypotonic in relation to the electrolytes (i.e., water is lost in excess of sodium and other electrolytes). The combination of hypotonic fluid loss and hyperglycemia leads to serum hyperosmolality. In turn, increased serum osmolality causes a shift of water from the cells. The net result is a loss of both intracellular fluid (ICF) and extracellular fluid (ECF), with individuals losing up to 25% of their total body water. Neurologic deficits (i.e., slowed mentation, confusion, seizures, coma) occur as a result of the altered CNS cell function from cell shrinkage.

As extracellular volume decreases, the blood becomes more viscous and its flow is impeded. Thromboemboli are common because of increased blood viscosity, enhanced platelet aggregation and adhesiveness, and patient immobility. Cardiac workload is increased and may lead to myocardial infarction (MI). Renal blood flow is decreased, potentially resulting in renal impairment or failure. Cerebrovascular accident may result from thromboemboli or decreased cerebral perfusion. These severe complications, in addition to the initial precipitating disorder, contribute to a mortality rate of 10% to 25%.

The onset of HHNK syndrome is often insidious and classically occurs in an older individual with type 2 DM who has a concomitant reduction in renal function. It is typically precipitated by some form of stress (e.g., infection, trauma, surgery) that increases the release of hormones (e.g., catecholamines, glucagon, cortisol), which raises blood glucose levels. The combination of hypovolemia and decreased renal function ultimately results in a rapid rise in blood glucose as a result of decreased urinary excretion of glucose. The mechanism responsible for the absence of elevated ketones is not fully understood, although it has been suggested that individuals with HHNK syndrome still produce enough insulin to maintain normal fat metabolism but that is insufficient for normal glucose use. The absence of ketoacidosis and the slow onset of vague neurologic symptoms in older adults often result in the initial misdiagnosis of HHNK syndrome as a primary neurologic disorder. (Table 20-1 provides a comparison of DKA and HHNK syndrome.)

## Potential Fluid, Electrolyte, and Acid-Base Disturbances

1. **Fluid volume deficit** caused by hyperglycemia-induced osmotic diuresis. Hypovolemia is treated with either isotonic saline (0.9% NaCl) or 0.45% saline solution. Fluid replacement is rapid: 1 to 2 liters (L) in the first hours of treatment, with 7 to 9 L total during the next 2 to 3 days (see Chapter 6).
2. **Hyponatremia** may be present initially because of the osmotic shift of water from the cells (pseudohyponatremia). The presence of hypertriglyceridemia may also contribute to pseudohyponatremia. In fact, glucose-induced osmotic diuresis causes a hypotonic fluid loss, with water lost in excess of sodium. If a patient's plasma sodium level on

Table 20-1   Comparison of DKA and HHNK syndrome

| Criterion | DKA | HHNK |
|---|---|---|
| Diabetes type | Usually type 1 | Usually type 2 |
| Typical age group | Any age | Usually > 50 years |
| History and risk factors | Undiagnosed type 1 DM; recent stressors such as surgery, trauma, infection, or MI; insufficient exogenous insulin | Undiagnosed type 2 DM; recent stressors such as surgery, trauma, pancreatitis, MI, or infection; high-caloric enteral or parenteral feedings in a compromised patient; use of diabetogenic drugs (e.g., phenytoin, thiazide diuretics, thyroid preparations, mannitol, corticosteroids, sympathomimetics) |
| Signs and symptoms | Polyuria, polydipsia, polyphagia, weakness, orthostatic hypotension, lethargy, changes in LOC, fatigue, nausea, vomiting, abdominal pain | Same as DKA, but with a slower onset and (commonly) predominant neurologic symptoms |
| Physical assessment | Dry and flushed skin, poor skin turgor, dry mucous membranes, decreased BP, tachycardia, altered LOC (e.g., irritability, lethargy, coma), Kussmaul's respirations, | Same as DKA, but no Kussmaul's respirations or fruity odor to the breath; instead, occurrence of tachypnea with shallow respirations |

| Monitoring parameters | *ECG:* Dysrhythmias associated with hyperkalemia (e.g., peaked T waves, widened QRS complex, prolonged PR interval, flattened or absent P wave); hypokalemia (potassium <3 mmol/L), which may produce depressed ST segments, flat or inverted T waves, or increased ventricular dysrhythmias | *ECG:* Evidence of hypokalemia as listed with DKA<br><br>*Hemodynamic measurements:* CVP >3 mm Hg below the patient's baseline; PADP and PAWP >4 mm Hg below the patient's baseline |
|---|---|---|
| Diagnostic tests | *Serum glucose:* 200-800 mg/dL<br>*Serum acetone:* Positive<br>*Urine glucose:* Positive<br>*Urine acetone:* "Large"<br>*Serum osmolality:* 300-350 mOsm/L<br>*Bicarbonate:* <5 mmol/L<br><br>*Serum pH:* <7.2<br>*Serum potassium:* Normal or elevated >5 mmol/L initially and then decreased | 800-2000 mg/dL<br>Usually absent<br>Positive<br>Negative<br>>350 mOsm/L<br>Normal or slightly decreased if mild acidosis present<br>Normal or mildly acidic (pH <7.4)<br>Normal or <3.5 mmol/L |

Modified from Horne MM: Endocrinologic dysfunctions. In Swearingen PL, Keen JH, editors: *Manual of critical care nursing: nursing interventions and collaborative management,* ed 4, St Louis, 2001, Mosby.

*BP,* Blood pressure; *BUN,* blood urea nitrogen; *CVA,* cerebrovascular accident; *CVP,* central venous pressure; *ECG,* electrocardiogram; *Hct,* hematocrit; *LOC,* level of consciousness; *mm Hg,* millimeters of mercury; *mmol/L,* millimoles/liter; *mOsm/L,* milliosmoles/liter; *PADP,* pulmonary artery diastolic pressure; *PAWP,* pulmonary artery wedge pressure; *WBC,* white blood cell count.

*Continued*

Table 20-1    Comparison of DKA and HHNK syndrome—cont'd

| Criterion | DKA | HHNK |
|---|---|---|
| | *Serum sodium:* Elevated, normal, or low | Elevated, normal, or low |
| | *Serum Hct:* Elevated because of osmotic diuresis with hemoconcentration | Elevated because of hemoconcentration |
| | *BUN:* Elevated > 20 mg/dL | Elevated |
| | *Serum creatinine:* > 1.5 mg/dL | Elevated |
| | *Serum phosphorus, magnesium, chloride:* Decreased | Decreased |
| | *WBC:* Elevated, even in the absence of infection | Normal unless infection present |
| Onset | Hours to days | Days to weeks |
| Mortality rate | < 10% | 10%-25% as a result of age group and complications such as CVA, thrombosis, and renal failure |

admission is normal or elevated, a massive water loss has occurred (see Chapter 7).

3. **Hypokalemia** caused by increased urinary losses from osmotic diuresis (see Chapter 8).

4. **Hypophosphatemia** caused by increased urinary losses from osmotic diuresis. Hypokalemia and hypophosphatemia are treated with a combination of IV potassium chloride and potassium phosphate (see Chapter 10).

5. **Hypomagnesemia** caused by increased urinary losses from osmotic diuresis (see Chapter 11).

6. **Metabolic** acidosis is usually mild if present; more significant acidosis may be caused by increased production and retention of lactic acid as a result of hypovolemia with tissue hypoxia. (A mild anion gap may be present with elevated lactate levels.) Acidosis usually resolves with treatment (insulin and fluids), but it may be treated with IV $NaHCO_3$ if severe (pH $< 7.10$), although this treatment is controversial (see Chapter 15).

## Diabetes Insipidus

Diabetes insipidus (DI) is caused either by a deficiency in the synthesis or release of antidiuretic hormone (ADH) from the posterior pituitary gland (neurogenic, or central, DI) or by a decrease in kidney responsiveness to ADH (nephrogenic DI), resulting in decreased water absorption by the renal tubules. Central DI may be idiopathic or may occur as a result of cerebral tumor, trauma, or hypoperfusion; it resolves with the administration of vasopressin (Table 20-2). In contrast, nephrogenic DI responds poorly to vasopressin and may be caused by a wide variety of medications and disorders, including electrolyte imbalance (e.g., hypokalemia, hypocalcemia).

Regardless of the cause, the individual with DI excretes large volumes of extremely dilute urine. As with DM, the cardinal symptoms of DI are polyuria and polydipsia. These remain the only symptoms as long as these individuals are able to drink and satisfy their thirst, thereby maintaining fluid volume. If the person is unable to access adequate amounts of water (e.g., an infant with congenital DI or the adult who is neurologically impaired), abnormal water loss results in a rapidly decreased ECF volume and increased serum sodium and

Table 20-2  Vasopressin preparations

| Generic Name | Trade Name | Onset | Duration | Usual Dosage | Advantages/ Disadvantages | Comments |
|---|---|---|---|---|---|---|
| Nasal | | | | | | |
| Vasopressin | Pitressin | Within 1 hour | 4-8 hours | 5-10 U bid-tid | Action decreased by nasal congestion/ discharge or atrophy of nasal mucosa | Administer with spray, cotton pledget, or dropper; used for chronic DI management |
| Desmopressin acetate | DDAVP* | Within 1 hour | 8-20 hours | 0.1-0.4 ml qd in 1-3 doses (10-40 μg) | See above | See above; stored in refrigerator at 4° C (39.2° F) |
| Lypressin | Diapid | Within 1 hour | 3-8 hours | 2-4 U qd (1-2 sprays) | See above | See above; stored at <40° C (100° F) |
| Subcutaneous | | | | | | |
| Vasopressin | Pitressin | ½-1 hour | 2-8 hours | 0.25-0.5 mL (5-10 U) q3-4 hours prn for increased thirst | | Typically used in acute care settings and for emergency |

| | | | | | | Kept refrigerated at 4° C (39.2° F) |
|---|---|---|---|---|---|---|
| Desmopressin DDAVP, acetate | Stimate | Within ½ hour | 1/2... hours | 0.5-1 mL (2-4 µg) qd in 2 divided doses | | |
| Intramuscular Vasopressin tannate in oil | Pitressin tannate in oil | Within 1-2 hours | 36-48 hours | 0.3-1 mL (1.5-5 U) q 2-3 days for increased thirst or increased urine output | Longer duration of action, with a slower absorption than the subcutaneous route; response cumulative over 2-3 days | Stored at 13° C-18° C (55° F-65° F) Shake well before withdrawing from vial; can warm solution with immersing vial in warm water |

From Horne MM: Endocrinologic dysfunctions. In Swearingen PL, Keen JH, editors: *Manual of critical care nursing: nursing interventions and collaborative management*, ed 4, St Louis, 2001, Mosby.

*Drug of choice.

*bid*, Twice a day; *DDAVP*, 1-deamino-8-D-arginine vasopressin; *prn*, as required; *q*, every; *qd*, every day; *tid*, three times a day; *U*, unit; *µg*, microgram.

*Continued*

Table 20-2  Vasopressin preparations—cont'd

| Generic Name | Trade Name | Onset | Duration | Usual Dosage | Advantages/ Disadvantages | Comments |
|---|---|---|---|---|---|---|
| Vasopressin tannate | Pitressin tannate | ½-1 hour | 2-8 hours | 0.25-0.5 mL (5-10 U) q 3-4 hours for increased thirst or increased urine output | Longer duration of action, which makes intramuscular forms more desirable for chronic management | |
| Intravenous | | | | | | |
| Desmopressin acetate | DDAVP | Within ½ hour | 1½-4 hours | 0.5-1 mL (2-4 µg) qd in 2 divided doses | Not for home use | Keep refrigerated at 4° C (39.2° F); dilute in 10-50 mL 0.9% NaCl and infuse over 15-30 minutes |

osmolality. Without treatment, severe ECF and ICF dehydration, hypotension, and shock can occur. Decreased cerebral perfusion and increased serum osmolality produce neurologic symptoms ranging from confusion, restlessness, and irritability to seizures and coma. The severity of and prognosis for DI vary with its cause. The onset may be sudden and dramatic, as with cerebral trauma, or it may be gradual, as with tumors or infiltrative disease.

## Potential Fluid, Electrolyte, and Acid-Base Disturbances

1. **Fluid volume deficit** caused by decreased water resorption by the renal tubule as a result of decreased ADH production or effectiveness. It is treated with hypotonic fluid replacement and correction of the cause (see Chapter 6).
2. **Hypernatremia** caused by increased free water loss as a result of decreased renal resorption of water. Hypernatremia also is corrected with hypotonic fluid replacement. Ironically, nephrogenic DI can be treated with diuretics such as thiazide that block the kidneys' ability to excrete free water (see Chapter 7).

# Syndrome of Inappropriate Secretion of Antidiuretic Hormone

Syndrome of inappropriate secretion of ADH (SIADH) develops as a result of excessive levels of circulating ADH. The causes of SIADH fall into one of three categories: (1) excessive production or release of ADH from CNS disorders such as meningitis or increased intracranial pressure; (2) respiratory disorders such as infections and lesions, which increase the release of ADH through an unknown mechanism; or (3) ectopic ADH secretion of malignant tumors, particularly oat cell carcinoma of the lung. In the presence of increased ADH, water that normally is excreted in the urine is inappropriately reabsorbed and returned to the circulation, diluting the serum sodium and decreasing serum osmolality. ECF volume expansion increases glomerular filtration and decreases the release of aldosterone, both of which act to increase urinary excretion of sodium, further reducing the serum sodium level. As the serum sodium level decreases, an osmotic gradient is created that favors an ICF shift. Increased ICF in the brain can result in cerebral edema with altered neurologic function and, ultimately, death if the condition is not treated.

SIADH typically is diagnosed on the basis of laboratory findings and patient history. Classic laboratory findings include serum hyponatremia and hypoosmolality, combined with inappropriately high urine sodium and osmolality. Treatment is aimed at correcting the primary problem, limiting water intake, and administering sodium. Medications such as lithium or demeclocycline (used for patients with malignant lung diseases), which inhibit the action of ADH on the renal tubule, may also be used. Furosemide may be given to increase diuresis and prevent pulmonary edema.

## Potential Fluid, Electrolyte, and Acid-Base Disturbances

1. **Hyponatremia** caused by excessive retention of water and continued urinary loss of sodium (see Chapter 7).
2. **Hypervolemia** caused by retention of water with cellular volume expansion (see Chapter 6).

NOTE: ECF volume expansion usually is minimized because of the decreased stimulus to aldosterone and increased stimulus to atrial natriuretic factor.

# Acute Adrenal Insufficiency

Adrenal insufficiency (decreased production of adrenocortical hormones) occurs as a result of either dysfunction of the adrenal glands (primary insufficiency) or inadequate stimulation of the adrenal glands by the anterior pituitary (secondary insufficiency). Conditions associated with primary adrenal insufficiency include autoimmune disease, infection (e.g., tuberculosis, AIDS, gram-negative sepsis), bilateral adrenal hemorrhage, bilateral adrenalectomy, tumor invasion, and enzymatic deficiencies. A decrease in the production of adrenocortical hormones because of a reduction in functioning adrenal tissue is also termed *Addison's disease*. Secondary adrenal insufficiency is associated with long-term exogenous steroid administration and destruction of the pituitary gland by tumors, infarcts, trauma, surgery, infection, or radiation therapy for intracranial lesions. Acute adrenal insufficiency (also known as *Addisonian crisis*) is a life-threatening condition characterized by severe fluid and electrolyte imbalances related to both mineralocorticoid and glucocorticoid deficiencies. Mineralocorticoid (aldosterone) deficiency results in large urinary losses of sodium and water with the development of hyponatremia and hypovolemia. In addition, hyperkalemia and metabolic acidosis can develop as the result of decreased urinary excretion of potassium and hydrogen. Glucocorticoid (cortisol) deficiency intensifies the clinical effects of hypovolemia by causing a decrease in vascular tone and decreased vascular response to catecholamines (epinephrine and norepinephrine). Cortisol depletion also may cause hypoglycemia because of the body's inability to maintain blood glucose levels in the fasting state. Severe hypotension, shock, and, eventually, death occur without adequate parenteral adrenocortical hormone and fluid replacement. For patients with chronic insufficiency, acute crises may be prevented by increasing replacement hormone doses during periods of stress.

## Potential Fluid, Electrolyte, and Acid-Base Disturbances

1. **Hypovolemia** caused by decreased resorption of sodium and water by the renal tubule as a result of the lack of aldosterone. It is treated with IV isotonic (0.9%) saline solution and IV hydrocortisone (see Chapter 6).
2. **Hyperkalemia** caused by decreased secretion and excretion of potassium by the renal tubule as a result of the lack of aldosterone. Hyperkalemia may be treated with Kayexalate (see Chapter 8).
3. **Metabolic acidosis** (usually mild), termed *type 4 renal tubular acidosis,* caused by decreased secretion and excretion of hydrogen by the renal tubule as a result of the lack of aldosterone. Hyperkalemia may contribute to the development of metabolic acidosis because it impairs ammonia ($NH_4$) production (see Chapter 15).
4. **Hyponatremia,** which may occur with chronic primary adrenocortical insufficiency because of hypovolemia-induced release of ADH with the retention of free water (see Chapter 7).

# Cardiac Disorders

# 21

## Congestive Heart Failure and Pulmonary Edema

Congestive heart failure (CHF) develops when the heart is unable to maintain a cardiac output sufficient to meet the metabolic needs of the tissues. Causes of CHF include coronary artery disease, hypertension, cardiomyopathy, and valvular disease. As the heart fails and the cardiac output drops, there is a reduction in effective circulating volume (ECV) with poor renal blood flow. This results in a reduction in the load of sodium and water filtered by the kidneys and stimulates the release of renin. Renin causes an increase in angiotensin II, a potent vasoconstrictor that increases systemic vascular resistance and the workload of the heart (afterload). Increased angiotensin II, in turn, leads to an increase in aldosterone, with retention of sodium and water by the kidneys and an increase in vascular volume (preload). Decreased ECV also stimulates the release of antidiuretic hormone (ADH), causing further retention of water by the kidneys. Because the diseased heart is unable to circulate this increased volume, the pressure within the venous circuit increases and edema develops.

When the left side of the heart is unable to pump the blood returning from the lungs into the systemic circulation, the hydrostatic pressure within the pulmonary circulation increases. If the hydrostatic pressure exceeds the pulmonary oncotic pressure, fluid leaks into the pulmonary interstitium, which results in pulmonary edema with impairment of oxygen exchange. Right ventricular failure usually occurs from left ventricular failure (the right heart must work harder as the pressure in the pulmonary vasculature increases), but it may occur independently in conditions such as cor pulmonale. When the right side of the heart fails, backup occurs in the venous circuit, with congestion of blood in body organs (e.g., liver, spleen) and edema formation.

## Potential Fluid, Electrolyte, and Acid-Base Disturbances

1. **Fluid volume excess** as evidenced by peripheral and pulmonary edema, caused by increased secretion of aldosterone and ADH. It is treated with diuretics and fluid and sodium restriction. Inotropic agents and vasodilators are administered to improve cardiac function (see Chapter 6).

2. **Hyponatremia** caused by increased secretion of ADH. (NOTE: ADH affects water retention only, whereas aldosterone causes retention of both sodium and water.) Hyponatremia resolves with fluid restriction and correction of the primary problem (see Chapter 7).

3. **Hypokalemia** caused by the use of potassium-wasting diuretics (e.g., furosemide). Furosemide is commonly used in the treatment of acute pulmonary edema because of its potent and rapid diuretic action when administered intravenously (IV) and its direct vasodilatory effect, which reduces preload (see Chapter 8).

4. **Respiratory alkalosis** may occur in pulmonary edema because of hypoxemia-induced hyperventilation (see Chapter 14).

5. **Respiratory acidosis** may develop if pulmonary edema is so severe that carbon dioxide retention occurs with hypoxemia (see Chapter 13).

6. **Metabolic acidosis** may develop as CHF worsens, leading to increased production of lactic acid by hypoxic tissues and decreased excretion of acids by the kidneys (see Chapter 15).

## Cardiogenic Shock

Shock is a state in which blood flow to peripheral tissue is inadequate for sustaining life. Usually cardiogenic shock is caused by a massive myocardial infarction (MI) that renders 40% or more of the myocardium dysfunctional as a result of ischemia or necrosis. As a result, cardiac output is reduced and all tissues suffer from inadequate perfusion. With decreased perfusion to the heart, coronary flow is reduced, impairing cardiac function, which further decreases cardiac output.

The first stage of shock is characterized by increased sympathetic discharge as the baroreceptors at the carotid sinus and aortic arch are stimulated by the drop in blood pressure.

The release of epinephrine and norepinephrine is a compensatory mechanism that increases cardiac output by increasing the heart rate and contractility of the uninjured myocardium. Vasoconstriction, a mechanism that increases blood pressure, also occurs. The second or middle stage of shock is characterized by decreased perfusion to the brain, kidneys, and heart. Lactate and pyruvic acid accumulate in the tissues, and metabolic acidosis occurs from anaerobic metabolism. In the late stage of shock, which is usually irreversible, compensatory mechanisms become ineffective and multiple organ failure occurs.

## Potential Fluid, Electrolyte, and Acid-Base Disturbances

1. **Fluid volume deficit** may be present because of prior diuretic therapy with potent diuretics (e.g., furosemide; see Chapter 6).

2. **Fluid volume excess** may be present or develop because of stimulation of the renin-angiotensin system, resulting in retention of sodium and water. Overly aggressive fluid therapy may be a contributing factor. Volume imbalances resolve with improved cardiac function (see Chapter 6).

3. **Hyponatremia** may be present from an increase in the release of ADH, resulting in retention of water (see Chapter 7).

4. **Metabolic acidosis** occurring with accumulation of lactate and pyruvic acid in the tissues as a result of decreased tissue perfusion. Severe metabolic acidosis (pH $< 7.10$) may necessitate treatment with IV sodium bicarbonate, although this treatment is controversial (see Chapter 15).

5. **If shock is prolonged,** the individual may have acute tubular necrosis (ATN) develop, which can lead to multiple fluid and electrolyte disturbances (see Chapter 22).

# Renal Failure

22

Renal failure (acute or chronic) may lead to a myriad of disturbances in fluid, electrolyte, and acid-base balance because the kidneys are the primary regulators of this balance. This is easy to appreciate after a review of the normal functions of the kidneys (Box 22-1).

Acute renal failure (ARF) is a sudden loss of renal function that may or may not be accompanied by oliguria. The kidneys lose the ability to maintain biochemical homeostasis, causing retention of metabolic waste and dramatic alterations in fluid, electrolyte, and acid-base balance. Although the alteration in renal function usually is reversible, ARF is associated with an overall mortality rate as high as 40%. However, the mortality rate varies greatly with the etiology of ARF, the patient's age, and any preexisting medical problems.

The causes of ARF are classified according to etiology as *prerenal, intrarenal,* and *postrenal* (Box 22-2). A decrease in renal function as a result of decreased renal perfusion but without renal parenchymal damage is termed *prerenal failure.* Causes of prerenal failure include fluid volume deficit, shock, and decreased cardiac function. If hypoperfusion has not been prolonged, restoration of renal perfusion restores normal renal function. A reduction in urine output that occurs because of obstruction to urine flow is termed *postrenal,* or *postobstructive, failure.* Conditions that cause postrenal failure include neurogenic bladder, tumors, and urethral strictures. Early detection of prerenal and postrenal failure is essential because, if prolonged, such failure can lead to parenchymal damage.

The most common cause of *intrarenal,* or *intrinsic, failure* (i.e., renal failure that develops from renal parenchymal damage) is acute tubular necrosis (ATN). Although typically associated with prolonged ischemia (prerenal failure) or exposure to nephrotoxins, ATN also can occur after transfusion

---

## Box 22-1 Functions of the Kidney

- Regulation of water and electrolyte balance. The kidneys play an important role in the regulation of sodium ion ($Na^+$), potassium ion ($K^+$), calcium ion ($Ca^{2+}$), magnesium ion ($Mg^{2+}$), hydrogen ion ($H^+$), chloride ion ($Cl^-$), phosphate ion ($PO_4^{3-}$), and bicarbonate ion ($HCO_3^-$).

- Maintenance of acid-base balance through the excretion of $H^+$ and the regeneration of $HCO_3^-$. As each $H^+$ is moved into the renal tubule to be excreted, an ion of $HCO_3^-$ is generated and returned to the extracellular fluid (ECF).

- Excretion of metabolic wastes (e.g., urea, uric acid, creatinine, unknown toxins).

- Excretion of foreign substances (e.g., medications, poisons, food additives).

- Production of the following:

  *Renin:* Helps regulate vascular volume and blood pressure through the regulation of $Na^+$ and water.

  *Erythropoietin:* Released in response to a low oxygen level in the renal cells; stimulates the production of red blood cells by the bone marrow.

  *Active form of vitamin D:* Increases the intestinal absorption of calcium, phosphorus, and magnesium; increases bone resorption (movement out) of calcium and phosphorus; and increases the resorption (saving) of calcium and phosphorus by the kidneys. The net result is that of helping maintain normal calcium, phosphorus, and magnesium levels.

  *Prostaglandins:* Primarily vasodilating substances; affect blood flow to and within the kidneys and increase kidney responsiveness to the effects of antidiuretic hormone (ADH) and aldosterone.

---

reactions, crushing injuries, or septic abortions. The clinical course of ATN is divided into three phases: oliguric (lasting approximately 7 to 21 days), diuretic (lasting 7 to 14 days), and recovery (which can continue for 3 to 12 months). Causes of intrarenal failure other than ATN include acute glomerulonephritis and malignant hypertension. (Box 22-3 provides a list

## Box 22-2  Causes of Acute Renal Failure

| Prerenal (Decreased Renal Perfusion) | Intrarenal (Parenchymal Damage; ATN) | Postrenal (Obstruction) |
|---|---|---|
| Fluid Volume Deficit | Nephrotoxic Agents | Calculi |
| ■ GI losses | ■ Antibiotics (e.g., aminoglycosides, sulfonamides, methicillin) | Tumor |
| ■ Hemorrhage | ■ Diuretics (e.g., furosemide) | Benign Prostatic Hypertrophy |
| ■ Third-space (interstitial) losses (e.g., burns, peritonitis) | ■ Contrast media | |
| ■ Dehydration from diuretic use | ■ Heavy metals (e.g., lead, gold, mercury) | Necrotizing Papillitis |
| | ■ Organic solvents (e.g., carbon tetrachloride, ethylene glycol) | Urethral Strictures |
| Hepatorenal Syndrome | | |
| Edema-Forming Conditions | Infection (gram-negative sepsis), Pancreatitis, and Peritonitis | Blood Clots |
| ■ Congestive heart failure | | Retroperitoneal Fibrosis |
| ■ Cirrhosis | | |
| ■ Nephrotic syndrome | Transfusion Reaction (hemolysis) | Neurogenic Bladder |

*Continued*

*IgA,* Immunoglobulin A.

## Box 22-2  Causes of Acute Renal Failure—cont'd

| Prenatal (Decreased Renal Perfusion) | Intrarenal (Parenchymal Damage; ATN) | Postrenal (Obstruction) |
|---|---|---|
| **Renal Vascular Disorders** <br> ■ Renal artery stenosis <br> ■ Renal artery thrombosis <br> ■ Renal vein thrombosis | **Rhabdomyolysis with Myoglobinuria** (severe muscle injury) <br> ■ Trauma (e.g., crush injuries) <br> ■ Exertion <br> ■ Seizures <br> ■ Drugs (e.g., heroin, barbiturates, intravenous amphetamines) <br><br> **Glomerular Diseases** <br> ■ Poststreptococcal glomerulonephritis <br> ■ IgA nephropathy (e.g., Berger's disease) <br> ■ Lupus glomerulonephritis <br> ■ Serum sickness <br> ■ Acute interstitial nephritis (drug-induced) <br><br> Ischemic Injury (prolonged prerenal) | |

**Box 22-3    Drugs That Necessitate Dosage Modification in Renal Failure**

| Antimicrobials | Cardiovascular Agents | Analgesics | Sedatives | Miscellaneous | Drugs to Avoid |
|---|---|---|---|---|---|
| Amikacin | Digoxin | Methadone | Phenobarbitol | Insulin | Tetracycline |
| Gentamicin | Procainamide | Morphine | Meprobamate | Cimetidine | Nitrofurantoin |
| Kanamycin | Guanethidine | | | Clofibrate | Spironolactone |
| Tobramycin | | | | Antacids ($Ca^{2+}$ aluminum salts)* | Amiloride |
| Amphotericin B | | | | | Aspirin |
| Vancomycin | | | | | Lithium carbonate |
| Lincomycin | | | | | Cisplatin |
| Sulfonamides | | | | | Nonsteroidal anti-inflammatory agents |
| Ethambutol | | | | | Magnesium-containing medications |
| Penicillins | | | | | Meperidine |
| | | | | | Glyburide |
| | | | | | Antacids ($Mg^{2+}$ salts) |

*$Ca^{2+}$ salts are the drugs of choice for phosphate binders.

of the most commonly used drugs that require dosage modification or avoidance for patients with ARF.)

Chronic renal failure (CRF) is a progressive, irreversible loss of renal function that develops over months to years. Eventually it can progress to end-stage renal disease (ESRD), at which time renal replacement therapy (dialysis or transplantation) is necessary to sustain life. Before ESRD occurs, the individual with CRF can lead a relatively normal life managed with diet and medications. The length of this period varies depending on the cause of renal failure and the patient's level of renal function at the time of diagnosis.

There are many causes of CRF, some of the most common being glomerulonephritis, diabetes mellitus, hypertension, and polycystic kidney disease. Regardless of the cause, the clinical presentation of CRF, particularly as an individual approaches ESRD, is similar. Retention of nitrogenous wastes and accompanying fluid and electrolyte imbalances adversely affect all body systems. Alterations in neuromuscular, cardiovascular, and gastrointestinal (GI) function are common. Renal osteodystrophy is an early and frequent complication. These collective manifestations of CRF are termed *uremia*.

## Potential Fluid, Electrolyte, and Acid-Base Disturbances

1. **Hypervolemia** caused by anuria or oliguria. It is treated with fluid restriction, diuretics, and, if necessary, dialysis (see Figs. 22-1 and 22-2 for depictions of dialysis; also see Chapter 6).

2. **Hypovolemia** during the diuretic phase of ARF because of excretion of large volumes of hypotonic urine, combined with existing fluid restriction. Hypovolemia also may occur in postrenal failure after release of the obstruction (postobstructive diuresis). Hypovolemia may be the precipitating event in prerenal failure (see Box 22-2 and Chapter 6).

3. **Hyponatremia** caused by excessive consumption or administration of hypotonic fluids (see Chapter 7).

4. **Hyperkalemia** caused by the kidneys' inability to excrete potassium and increased tissue catabolism with the release of intracellular potassium. Hyperkalemia is managed with a combination of dietary restrictions and removal via cation exchange resins (Kayexalate) or dialysis. Acute life-threatening hyperkalemia may be temporarily corrected with the

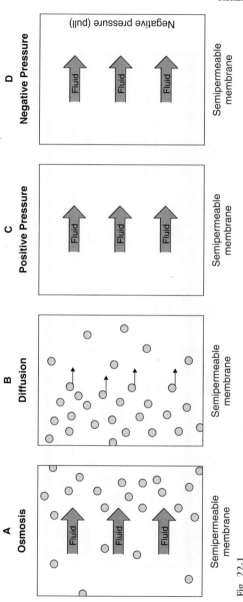

Fig. 22-1
Dialysis is based on principles of osmosis (A), diffusion (B), and ultrafiltration. Ultrafiltration occurs when either positive pressure (C) or negative pressure (D) is placed on the system. Ultrafiltration can be maximized by simultaneously exerting both positive and negative pressure on the system.
(From Phipps WJ, Monahan FD, Sands JK et al: *Medical-surgical nursing: health and illness perspectives*, ed 7, St Louis, 2003, Mosby.)

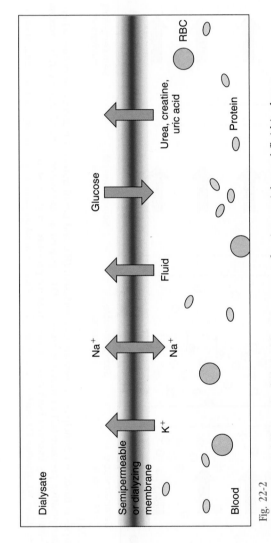

Fig. 22-2
Osmosis and diffusion in dialysis. Net movement of major particles and fluid is shown. (From Phipps WJ, Monahan FD, Sands JK et al: *Medical-surgical nursing: health and illness perspectives*, ed 7, St Louis, 2003, Mosby.)

administration of glucose and insulin or sodium bicarbonate (see Chapter 8).

5. **Hypokalemia** during the diuretic phase of ARF, especially in a patient with potassium restriction (see Chapter 8).

6. **Hyperphosphatemia** caused by the kidneys' inability to excrete phosphorus. It is treated with limiting dietary intake of high-phosphorus foods and administration of phosphorus-binding medications (see Chapter 10).

7. **Hypocalcemia** caused by decreased levels of the metabolically active form of vitamin D, hyperphosphatemia (NOTE: Calcium and phosphorus have a reciprocal relationship; as one increases, the other tends to decrease), skeletal resistance to parathyroid hormone (PTH) (the hormone released by the parathyroid gland in response to a low serum calcium level), and hypoalbuminemia. Treatment begins with regulation of phosphorus via phosphorous-binding medications. Later, vitamin D replacement and additional calcium supplements may be necessary (see Chapter 9).

8. **Hypermagnesemia** caused by the kidneys' inability to excrete magnesium. Hypermagnesemia usually can be prevented with avoiding magnesium-containing medications and supplements (see Chapter 11).

9. **Metabolic acidosis** caused by the kidneys' inability to excrete the body's daily load of nonvolatile acids. Limiting dietary intake of protein and preventing tissue catabolism help minimize acidosis. Dialysis provides some buffer replacement through the addition of bicarbonate or acetate to the dialysate (see Figs. 22-1 and 22-2 for depictions of dialysis; also see Chapter 15).

# Acute
# Pancreatitis

23

Acute pancreatitis is a potentially life-threatening condition caused by abnormal activation of pancreatic enzymes. A variety of conditions are associated with pancreatitis, including trauma and infection; however, the most common are chronic alcoholism and biliary tract disease (Box 23-1). Although the exact pathogenesis is unknown, injury to acinar cells results in the release and activation of pancreatic enzymes, causing autodigestion of the gland. Damage to the pancreas can range from acute edema to necrosis and hemorrhage. An individual with acute pancreatitis has acute abdominal pain and tenderness that may be precipitated by a meal or heavy alcohol intake. Nausea, weakness, ileus, diaphoresis, tachycardia, and hypotension often are present. Laboratory findings include elevated levels of serum amylase, serum lipase, and urine amylase and decreased levels of serum calcium and serum albumin.

Several potentially severe complications may accompany acute pancreatitis. The most common complication is intravascular fluid (IVF) volume deficit as a result of loss of fluid into the interstitium and retroperitoneum. Release of vasoactive amines results in increased capillary permeability, vasodilation, and depressed myocardial function. Hypoalbuminemia and hemorrhage from rupture of necrotic pancreatic vessels also may contribute to intravascular volume loss. Hypovolemia and hypotension, in turn, can lead to the development of prerenal acute renal failure (ARF) and shock. Other severe complications include respiratory failure, rupture of abscessed pancreatic pseudocytes, and tetany from severe hypocalcemia.

## Potential Fluid, Electrolyte, and Acid-Base Disturbances

1. **Fluid volume deficit** caused by loss of fluid into the interstitium and retroperitoneum, vomiting, gastric suction, diarrhea, diaphoresis, and hemorrhage. Hypovolemia is

## Box 23-1 Etiologies of Acute Pancreatitis

Toxins and Metabolic Factors

- Ethanol (i.e., alcoholism)
- Hypertriglyceridemia
- Hypercalcemia (e.g., hyperparathyroidism)
- Renal failure
- Cystic fibrosis

Structural and Mechanical Factors

- Trauma
- Gallstones (i.e., biliary tract disease)
- Spasm sphincter of Oddi (i.e., biliary tract disease)

Infection

- Bacterial,* viral, or parasitic
- Tuberculosis
- Mumps

Ischemic Factors

- Severe, prolonged shock
- Vasculitis
- Atherosclerosis

Drugs

- Sulfonamides
- Thiazide diuretics and furosemide
- Estrogens (e.g., oral contraceptives)
- Tetracycline
- Pentamidine
- Azathioprine

Other Specific Precipitating Events

- Endoscopic retrograde cholangiopancreatography (ERC)
- Hypothermia
- Peptic ulcer
- Inflammatory bowel disease
- Neoplasms
- Post organ transplant
- Pregnancy (third trimester)
- Postoperative state

*Most common infection.

primarily treated with crystalloids, although colloids (e.g., albumin) may be added. A large volume of parenteral fluids is necessary if shock is present. No oral fluids are administered until the patient is pain free and has bowel sounds. Calcium, potassium, and magnesium are added to intravenous (IV) fluids as needed (see Chapter 6).

2. **Hyponatremia** may develop because of a loss of sodium-containing fluids, accompanied by a hypovolemia-induced increase in antidiuretic hormone (ADH) secretion (see Chapter 7).

3. **Hypocalcemia** caused by calcium deposition in areas of fat necrosis, decreased secretion of parathyroid hormone (PTH; NOTE: PTH is the primary regulator of serum calcium levels.), hypoalbuminemia, and ARF (if it develops). Serum $Ca^{++}$ values of less than 8 milligrams/deciliter (mg/dl) are not uncommon. IV calcium gluconate is indicated for the treatment of significant or symptomatic hypocalcemia (see Chapter 9).

4. **Hypomagnesemia** caused by abnormal gastrointestinal (GI) losses and deposition of magnesium in areas of fat necrosis (see Chapter 11).

5. **Hypokalemia** caused by abnormal GI losses (see Chapter 8).

6. **Respiratory alkalosis** may develop in a patient with respiratory complications because of hypoxemia-induced hyperventilation (see Chapter 14).

7. **Parenteral feeding** is indicated for patients with severe pancreatitis (see Chapter 26).

# Hepatic Failure

# 24

Hepatic failure is a severe loss of liver function that may develop rapidly, as with viral or drug-induced hepatitis (Box 24-1), or slowly, as with Laennec's cirrhosis. In the pediatric population, it may also occur as the result of Reye's syndrome or genetic disorders. As liver insufficiency progresses, normal functions of the liver, such as nutrient, hormone, and bilirubin metabolism, are lost. The liver is no longer able to metabolize bilirubin, leading to increased bilirubin levels that result in jaundice and a deficiency of the fat soluble vitamins A, D, and K. Lack of adequate vitamin K, combined with decreased hepatic production of several clotting factors, decreased clearance of activated clotting factors, and thrombocytopenia, results in the bleeding tendency that is common in persons with hepatic failure. Decreased synthesis of albumin in conjunction with intrahepatic vascular obstruction contributes to the development of ascites and decreased intravascular volume (see the discussion in Chapter 6). Reduced vascular volume stimulates the release of renin, angiotensin, aldosterone, and antidiuretic hormone (ADH), which collectively act on the kidneys to conserve sodium and water, potentiating the development of ascites and contributing to peripheral edema.

Loss of liver function results in dysfunction in other organs such as the brain, the lungs, and the kidneys. The damaged liver is unable to metabolize substances such as ammonia, which are toxic to the brain. Although the exact pathogenesis of hepatic encephalopathy remains unclear, elevated ammonia levels are associated with worsening encephalopathy. Hepatorenal syndrome, a type of acute renal failure (ARF) that develops with advanced hepatic disease, is believed to develop because of unopposed renal vasoconstriction as a result of chronic release of renin, ADH, and norepinephrine. Decreased hepatic synthesis of prostaglandin precursors may limit normal renal

| Box 24-1    Drugs with Hepatotoxic Potential |
|---|

| Predictable Reaction | Nonpredicatable/ Idiosyncratic Reaction |
|---|---|
| ■ Acetaminophen | ■ Allopurinol |
| ■ Carbon tetrachloride | ■ Anabolic steroids |
| ■ Cholecystographic dyes | ■ Chlorpromazine |
| ■ Ethanol | ■ Chlorpropamide |
| ■ Halothane | ■ Clindamycin |
| ■ L-Asparaginase | ■ Erythromycin |
| ■ Methotrexate | ■ Imipramine |
| ■ Mithramycin | ■ Isoniazid |
| ■ Mushroom poisoning | ■ Methyldopa |
| ■ Puromycin | ■ Monamine oxidase |
| ■ Rifamycin | (MAO) inhibitors |
| ■ Tetracycline | ■ Oral contraceptives |
| ■ Urethane | ■ Oxacillin |
| ■ 6-Mercaptopurine | ■ Phenytoin |
|  | ■ Sulfonamides |

Modified from Phipps WJ, Monahan FD, Sands JK et al: *Medical-surgical nursing: health and illness perspectives,* ed 7, St Louis, 2003, Mosby.

protective mechanisms. Circulatory changes also occur in the lungs with the development of a significant ventilation-perfusion mismatch. Hyperventilation and respiratory alkalosis are also common.

## Potential Fluid, Electrolyte, and Acid-Base Disturbances

1. **Alterations in fluid volume** may be present as evidenced by ascites and peripheral edema. Ascites occurs in cirrhosis because of hepatic venous obstruction and retention of sodium and water by the kidneys, which together increase the hydrostatic pressure in the sinusoids, favoring movement of fluid into the peritoneal space. The increased sodium and water retention that occurs with ascites is believed to be caused by both abnormal handling of sodium and water by the kidneys (the overflow, or overfill, theory) and compensatory retention of sodium and water caused by a reduction in effective circulating volume (ECV) that stimulates the

renin-aldosterone system (the underfill theory). Reduction in ECV is the result of decreased hepatic synthesis of albumin (NOTE: Albumin helps hold the vascular volume in the vascular space.), peripheral vasodilation, and ascites formation itself. An increase in pressure within the peritoneal cavity caused by ascites results in increased femoral venous pressure. This, combined with hypoalbuminemia, leads to the development of peripheral edema. Edema and ascites may be treated with fluid and sodium restriction and potassium-sparing diuretics. Because salt retention is sustained by hyperaldosteronism, diuretics that affect the distal tubule are preferred. The most commonly used potassium-sparing diuretics for this purpose are spironolactone, triamterene, and amiloride. Potassium-wasting diuretics usually are avoided because of the risk of hypokalemic metabolic alkalosis, although furosemide may be added cautiously to spironolactone to increase diuresis. Massive or tense ascites may necessitate paracentesis. Refractory ascites may necessitate placement of a percutaneous transjugular intrahepatic portosystemic shunt (TIPS). The TIPS provides communication between the hepatic vein and the portal vein and aids in decreasing ascites, although the exact mechanism is not fully understood. (See Chapter 6 for a discussion of hypervolemia, edema, and diuretics.) NOTE: Intravascular hypovolemia may develop with excessive use of diuretics or rapid removal of ascitic fluid.

2. **Hyponatremia** is common in patients with cirrhosis with ascites and edema, especially in the terminal stage. Hyponatremia is dilutional and is the result of abnormal renal handling of water (see Chapter 7).

3. **Hypokalemia** is commonly seen in patients with cirrhosis with ascites and edema. Causes of hypokalemia in these individuals include poor dietary intake, administration of potassium-wasting diuretics, elevated aldosterone levels (aldosterone causes an increased urinary excretion of potassium), magnesium depletion (hypomagnesemia often is associated with hypokalemia), and vomiting. NOTE: Hypokalemia may cause an increase in serum ammonia levels and precipitate hepatic coma. Use of potassium-sparing diuretics helps prevent hypokalemia (see Chapter 8).

4. **Hyperkalemia** may occur when the liver disease is complicated by renal failure, inappropriate use of potassium-sparing diuretics, or overuse of salt substitutes. (See Chapter 6 for a discussion of diuretic therapy; also see Chapter 8.)

5. **Hypocalcemia** may occur with alcoholic cirrhosis as the result of poor oral intake or magnesium depletion (hypomagnesemia causes a reduction in the release and action of parathyroid hormone [PTH]; see Chapter 10).

6. **Hypomagnesemia** may occur with alcoholic cirrhosis because of poor oral intake, decreased gastrointestinal (GI) absorption, abnormal GI losses, and increased urinary excretion (see Chapter 11).

7. **Hypophosphatemia** occurs with chronic alcoholism, especially during acute withdrawal, as a result of poor dietary intake, increased GI losses with vomiting and diarrhea, use of phosphorus-binding antacids, hyperventilation (respiratory alkalosis causes an intracellular shift of phosphorus), and increased urinary losses (see Chapter 10).

8. **Respiratory alkalosis** may occur with all types of liver disease as the result of direct stimulation of the medullary respiratory center. Rapid shallow breathing may also be a result of abdominal pressure from ascites impairing lung expansion. Positioning in a semi-Fowler's position may allow free diaphragmatic movement with improved lung expansion. Alkalosis increases the cellular uptake of ammonia and, combined with hypokalemia, may precipitate hepatic coma (see Chapter 14).

9. **Respiratory acidosis** may occur as ascites increases and further impairs free movement of the diaphragm and lung expansion. (A semi-Fowler's position may allow improved lung expansion.) Intubation may be necessary if encephalopathy is present and respiratory status declines further. Careful monitoring of respiratory status is essential because hypoxemia can worsen encephalopathy.

10. **Metabolic alkalosis** also may occur with liver failure as a result of diuretic therapy. (See Chapter 6 for a discussion of metabolic alkalosis and diuretic therapy; also see Chapter 16.)

11. **Metabolic acidosis** may develop with severe chronic liver disease because of the liver's inability to metabolize lactic acid, the presence of alcoholism-induced and starvation-induced ketoacidosis, renal failure with the retention of acids, and the loss of bicarbonate in diarrhea (see Chapter 15).

# Burns

# 25

The skin is a complex organ that provides the body's first line of defense against a potentially hostile environment. It protects against infection, prevents the loss of body fluids, helps control body temperature, functions as an excretory and sensory organ, aids in activating vitamin D, and influences body image. Burns are a common, yet largely preventable, form of skin injury. In the initial phase of thermal injury, marked shifts in fluids and electrolytes pose the greatest risk to recovery. The immediate goal of therapy for major burns is preservation of vital organ function in the presence of significant hypovolemia and acidosis. The challenge of treatment is to maintain vascular volume and tissue perfusion with a minimum of edema formation.

In burns that cover less than 30% of the body, fluid shifts are limited to the area of the burn injury. Injured tissues release chemical mediators that increase local capillary permeability, allowing both colloids and crystalloids to move into the interstitial space. Increased capillary permeability is greatest during the first 8 to 12 hours after the burn, although full recovery of capillary integrity does not occur for 2 to 3 days. When burns cover more than 30% of the body, fluid shifts occur in both burned and nonburned tissue. The edema that develops in nonburned tissue is believed to be caused largely by hypoproteinemia resulting from a loss of protein into the burned tissue and to a lesser extent by the action of circulating vasoactive substances. In addition, thermal injury decreases cell membrane potential, allowing sodium and water to enter the cells, causing cellular swelling. The loss of skin also leads to a direct loss of fluid and heat from the body. Metabolic acidosis develops because of decreased tissue perfusion. Inhalation injury or injury to the upper airways with development of tissue edema limits the ability of the lungs to compensate for metabolic acidosis via hyperventilation. Severe inhalation injury may lead to profound hypoxemia and respiratory acidosis, which necessitate mechanical ventilation.

Burns are classified according to wound depth and are described as *superficial, partial-thickness,* or *full-thickness burns,* depending on the layer of skin involved. Partial-thickness burns, which involve the epidermis, may be either superficial (i.e., dry, without blisters and edema) or deep (i.e., moist, with blisters, blebs, and edema, involving the epidermis and varying levels of the dermis). Full-thickness burns destroy all epidermal elements and may involve subcutaneous fat, connective tissue, and bone. Skin grafting is necessary if the burns are larger than 4 centimeters (cm) in diameter (Table 25-1 lists the characteristics of the various types of burns).

One of the first steps in burn therapy is to determine the extent of the burn wound (Figs. 25-1 and 25-2) and the magnitude of the burn injury (Table 25-2). Burn magnitude and severity determine whether the patient needs transfer to a specialized burn center for treatment (Table 25-3 lists factors that determine burn severity). Knowledge of the extent of the burn wound is essential in estimating the volume of fluid needed to replace what has been lost into the tissues.

Aggressive fluid replacement is necessary during the initial resuscitation phase. Several formulas advocating the use of both crystalloids and colloids have been developed to direct fluid therapy (Table 25-4). Some formulas recommend crystalloids for the first 24 hours with a switch primarily to colloids on the second day. Others recommend the use of both crystalloids and colloids during the first 24 hours after the burn. In either case, the key to effective treatment is the tailoring of fluid therapy to the individual's needs and response to fluid replacement.

Mobilization of edema begins at approximately 72 hours after the burn. Intravascular fluid (IVF) overload with congestive heart failure is a risk at this time. Because the body must rid itself of excess fluid that was necessary during the initial acute phase, massive diuresis of fluid is expected, and this loss should not be replaced fully. Careful monitoring of hemodynamic status is essential during this phase to prevent dangerous fluid volume changes.

Table 25-1 Burn wound classification

| Degree of Burn | Cause of Injury | Depth of Injury | Wound Characteristics | Treatment Course |
|---|---|---|---|---|
| First-degree burn | Prolonged ultraviolet light exposure; brief exposure to hot liquids | Limited damage to epithelium; skin intact | Erythematous, hypersensitive, no blister formation | Complete healing within 3 to 5 days without scarring |
| Superficial partial-thickness burn (second-degree) | Brief exposure to flash, flame, or hot liquids | Epidermis destroyed; minimal damage to superficial layers of dermis; epidermal appendages intact | Moist and weepy, pink or red, blisters, blanching, hypersensitive | Complete healing within 21 days with minimal or no scarring |
| Deep partial-thickness burn (second-degree) | Intense radiant energy; scalding liquids, semi-liquids (e.g., tar), or solids; flame | Epidermis destroyed; underlying dermis damaged; some epidermal appendages remain intact | Pale, decreased moistness, blanching absent or prolonged, intact sensation to deep pressure but not to pinprick | Prolonged healing (often longer than 21 days); may necessitate skin grafting to achieve complete healing with better |

| | | | | Necessitates skin grafting |
|---|---|---|---|---|
| Full-thickness burn (third-degree) | Prolonged contact with flame or scalding liquids; steam; hot objects; chemicals; electrical current | Epidermis, dermis, and epidermal appendages destroyed; injury through dermis | Dry, leathery, pale, mottled brown, or red; thrombosed vessels visible; insensate | Necessitates skin grafting |
| Full-thickness burn (fourth-degree) | Electrical current; prolonged contact with flame (e.g., an unconscious victim) | Epidermis, dermis, and epidermal appendages destroyed; injury involves connective tissue, muscle, and possibly bone | Dry; charred or mottled brown, white, or red; no sensation; limited or no movement of involved extremities or digits | Necessitates skin grafting; amputation of involved extremities or digits likely |

From Carrougher GJ: Burn wound assessment and topical treatment. In Carrougher GJ: *Burn care and therapy*, St Louis, 1998, Mosby.

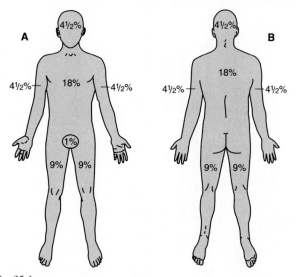

Fig. 25-1
Estimation of adult burn injury: rule of nines. **A,** Anterior view.
**B,** Posterior view.
(From Thompson JM, McFarland GK, Hirsch JE et al: *Mosby's clinical nursing,*
ed 5, St Louis, 2002, Mosby.)

## Potential Fluid, Electrolyte, and Acid-Base Disturbances

1. **Hypovolemia** caused by increased capillary permeability,
   with loss of IVF and proteins into the interstitium and
   evaporative loss of fluid through the burn wound. The
   plasma-to-interstitial fluid (ISF) shift occurs during the
   first 2 to 3 days. Later, there is a shift of fluid from
   the interstitium back into the plasma. **Hypervolemia** may
   develop at this time, especially if there has been aggressive
   fluid replacement during the initial phase. As discussed,
   fluid replacement may involve the use of both crystalloids
   (usually lactated Ringer's solution) and colloids (usually
   albumin). Hypertonic sodium chloride (NaCl) solutions
   have been advocated by some burn centers (see Chapter 6).
2. **Hyponatremia** caused by a hypovolemia-induced increase
   in antidiuretic hormone (ADH). A NaCl solution is administered to maintain the serum sodium level within an

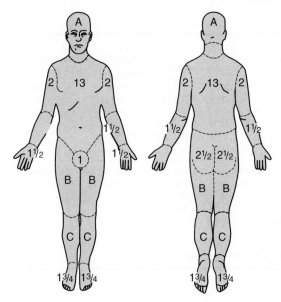

Relative percentages of areas affected by growth
(age in years)

|  | 0 | 1 | 5 | 10 | 15 | Adult |
|---|---|---|---|---|---|---|
| Half of head | 9½ | 8½ | 6½ | 5½ | 4½ | 3½ |
| Half of thigh | 2¾ | 3¼ | 4 | 4¼ | 4½ | 4¾ |
| Half of leg | 2½ | 2½ | 2¾ | 3 | 3¼ | 3½ |

Second degree _____ and
Third degree _____ =
Total percent burned\_\_\_\_

Fig. 25-2

Estimation of adult burn injury: Lund and Browder chart. Areas
designated by letters (*A, B,* and *C*) represent percentages of
body surface area that vary according to age. The accompanying table indicates relative percentages of these areas at
various stages in life.

(From Sabiston DC Jr, editor: *Textbook of surgery: the biological basis of modern
surgical practice,* ed 11, Philadelphia, 1977, WB Saunders. In Thompson JM,
McFarland GK, Hirsch JE et al: *Mosby's clinical nursing,* ed 5, St Louis, 2002,
Mosby.)

Table 25-2     American Burn Association classification system

| Magnitude of Burn Injury | Partial-Thickness | | Full Thickness Adults and Children (% TBSA) | Special Location* | Complications (Poor Risk, Fractures, and Other Trauma) |
|---|---|---|---|---|---|
| | Adult (% TBSA) | Children (% TBSA) | | | |
| Major | >25% | >20% | >10% | + | + |
| Moderate | 15%-25% | 10%-20% | 2%-10% | − | − |
| Minor | <15% | <10% | <2% | − | − |

Modified from Johnson J: Burns. In Swearingen PL, Keen JH, editors: *Manual of critical care nursing: nursing interventions and collaborative management,* ed 4, St Louis, 2001, Mosby.
*Hands, face, eyes, ears, feet, and genitalia.
*TBSA,* Total body surface area.

Table 25-3     Factors that determine burn severity

| Criterion | Factors |
|---|---|
| Extent | Severity depends on intensity and duration of exposure |
| Depth | Severity depends on intensity and duration of exposure |
| Age | Patients <2 years and >60 years |
| Medical history | Preexisting conditions (e.g., heart disease, chronic renal failure) |
| Body part | Special burn areas: hands, face, eyes, ears, feet, and genitalia |
| Complications | Burns with concomitant trauma (e.g., fractures) |

From Johnson J: Burns. In Swearingen PL, Kenn JH, editors: *Manual of critical care nursing: nursing interventions and collaborative management,* ed 4, St Louis, 2001, Mosby.

acceptable range. Pseudohypernatremia from hemoconcentration may be seen in the early phase of treatment if evaporative losses are not adequately replaced (see Chapter 7).
3. **Hyperkalemia** caused by release of potassium from damaged cells. This most likely occurs when the burn injury

Table 25-4 Adult burn resuscitation formulas

| Formula Name | Recommended Solutions | Formula for Estimating Fluid Needs |
|---|---|---|
| **Initial 24 Hours after Injury** | | |
| Evans* | 0.9% Normal saline plus colloid solution | 1 mL/kg/% TBSA burn<br>1 mL/kg/% TSBA burn |
| Brooke* | Lactated Ringer's solution plus colloid solution | 1.5 mL/kg/% TBSA burn<br>0.5 mL/kg/% TBSA burn |
| Hypertonic saline (Monafo) | $Na^+$ 250 mmol/L | Volume to maintain urine output at 30 mL/hour |
| Modified Brooke* | Lactated Ringer's solution | 2 mL/kg/% TBSA burn |
| Parkland* | Lactated Ringer's solution | 4 mL/kg/% TBSA burn |

From Gordon MD, Winfree JH: Fluid resuscitation after a major burn. In Carrougher GJ: *Burn care and therapy*, St Louis, 1998, Mosby.
*The total estimated volume is calculated, with half administered over the initial 8 hours after injury and the remaining half over the subsequent 16 hours.

*Continued*

Table 25-4   Adult burn resuscitation formulas—cont'd

| Formula Name | Recommended Solutions | Formula for Estimating Fluid Needs |
|---|---|---|
| **Second 24 Hours after Injury** | | |
| Evans | 0.9% Normal saline plus 5% dextrose in water | 50% of first 24-hour requirement 2000 mL |
| Brooke | Lactated Ringer's solution plus 5% dextrose in water | 50%-75% of first 24-hour fluid requirement 2000 mL |
| Hypertonic saline | 33% Isotonic salt solution | 0.6 mL/kg/% TBSA burn plus replacement of insensible losses |
| Modified Brooke | Colloid solution (diluted to physiologic concentration) plus 5% dextrose in water | 0.3-0.5 mL/kg/% TBSA burn (0.3 mL/kg/% TBSA burn for injuries of 30%-50%; up to 0.5 mL/kg/% TBSA burn for injuries > 50% TBSA) Volume to maintain desired urine output |
| Parkland | 25% Albumin plus 5% dextrose in water | 20%-60% of calculated plasma volume Volume to maintain desired urine output |

is complicated by acute renal failure. **Hypokalemia** may develop during the recovery phase because of a shift of potassium back into the cells, increased tissue utilization of potassium as wounds heal, and increased excretion of potassium in the urine (see Chapter 8).

4. **Hypocalcemia** may develop because of a loss of extracellular fluid (ECF) from the burn wound and a shift of calcium to the wound (see Chapter 9).

5. **Hypophosphatemia** commonly is associated with burns and occurs several days after the burn injury. The exact cause is unknown, but it may occur because of elevated calcitonin levels or respiratory alkalosis (see Chapter 10).

6. **Metabolic acidosis** may occur because of the release of acids from damaged tissue and the production of lactic acid if hypovolemia has led to shock. Metabolic acidosis can be avoided or minimized with early treatment of fluid volume deficit (see Chapter 15).

7. **Respiratory alkalosis** may develop because of hyperventilation from pain and anxiety. After resuscitation (if no inhalation injury is present), hyperventilation at two times the normal minute ventilation is common and is associated with mild hypoxemia during edema resorption (see Chapter 14).

8. **Respiratory acidosis** may develop with severe inhalation injury or as a result of restricted chest wall movement from edema development under eschar on the lateral and anterior chest wall (see Chapter 13).

# Providing Nutritional Support

## 26

The balance between nutrient intake and nutrient requirements determines nutritional status. The goals of nutritional therapy are to meet daily nutritional needs, replete any nutritional deficiencies, prevent further protein-calorie malnutrition, and promote a state of optimal nutritional status. For patients with fluid, electrolyte, and nutritional disturbances, the nurse's role is not only to assist with identification and implementation of interventions for patients but also to evaluate the effectiveness of the prescribed interventions and to communicate with other healthcare team members regarding these findings.

## Nutritional Assessment

Because no single sensitive and comprehensive tool exists to assess a patient's nutritional status, multiple sources of information are used. These include a patient's historical data, nutritional history, physical examination, anthropometric data, and biochemical data.

### Medical History

The medical record is reviewed to obtain information on factors that affect a patient's nutritional status or therapy. Data obtained include acute or chronic diseases, nutritional diagnoses/deficiencies, medical interventions, surgeries, medications, weight changes, psychosocial issues, or any other information that provides insight into nutritional care. This information helps determine the most appropriate route or method of nutritional therapy and the specific formulations and amounts that optimize nutritional care.

## Nutritional History

A nutritional history is compiled to reveal the adequacy of usual and recent dietary intake. A nurse must be alert to excesses or deficiencies of nutrients, restricted eating patterns or diets, or excessive supplementation. Anything that impairs adequate selection, preparation, ingestion, digestion, absorption, or excretion of nutrients should be noted. If a patient is determined to be at risk nutritionally, pursue a referral to a dietitian to allow for more in-depth nutritional evaluation if available. The following may be included in a nutritional history:

- A review of the patient's usual dietary intake; may be obtained with a 3- or 7-day diet history, food frequency questionnaire, or 24-hour recall
- Dietary influences from ethnic, cultural, or religious practices
- Any food allergies, intolerances, or aversions
- Use of nutritional supplements, including nonconventional or herbal supplements
- Recent weight gain or loss
- Chewing or swallowing difficulties; condition of teeth
- Changes in appetite or satiety level
- Nausea, vomiting, or pain with eating
- Altered pattern of elimination (e.g., constipation, diarrhea, excessive or altered ostomy output)
- Use of medications that affect nutritional requirements or the digestion, use, or excretion of nutrients
- Excessive alcohol consumption
- Social situations/physical limitations that hinder ability to obtain and prepare food

## Physical Examination

Most physical findings are not conclusive for a particular nutritional deficiency. However, the following may be indicative of nutritional inadequacies and should be noted:

- Abnormalities in skin integrity, lips/tongue/mucosa, eyes, hair, or nails
- Impaired wound healing
- Loss of muscle and adipose stores

▪ Loss of strength or endurance

Current assessment findings should be compared with past assessments.

## Anthropometric Data

Anthropometrics is the measurement of the body or its parts.

**Height:** Used to determine appropriateness of weight and to calculate body mass index (BMI) and is factored into predictive energy equations. If a patient's height is unavailable or impossible to measure with standing, an estimate can be obtained from the patient's family or significant other or by measuring the sum of body parts, measuring knee-height and converting to height via appropriate equations, measuring arm span (from tip of middle fingers with arms fully extended; this measurement is equivalent to height), or comparing the patient's recumbent length with the known length of the mattress.

**Weight:** A readily available and practical indicator of nutritional status that can be factored into predictive energy equations or used to calculate BMI. Nutritional status can be stratified into level of malnutrition with weight comparisons with previous, usual, or desirable weight. Changes may be reflective of fluid retention, diuresis, dehydration, surgical resections, traumatic amputations, or the weight of dressings or equipment and should be interpreted appropriately for any of these circumstances. It is helpful to remember that 1 liter (L) of fluid equals 1 kilogram (kg) or approximately 2 pounds (lb). Ideal or desirable body weight for adults is commonly determined with the Hamwi method:

Males: 106 lb for the first 5 feet (ft); add 6 lb per inch over 5 ft. Females: 100 lb for the first 5 ft; add 5 lb per inch over 5 ft. This weight is adjusted 10% less for small frames or 10% more for large frames.

**Body mass index:** Used to evaluate the weight of adults. One calculation and one set of standards are applicable to both men and women.

$$\text{BMI (kg/m}^2) = \frac{\text{Weight (kg)}}{\text{Height (m)} \times \text{Height (m)}}$$

To convert pounds and inches to metric measurements, use the following formulas:

    Divide pounds by 2.2 to convert to kilograms.

    Multiply inches by 2.54 to convert to centimeters.

    Divide inches by 39.37 to convert to meters.

BMI values of 19 to 27 are optimal. Values greater than 27 indicate obesity, and values less than 19 indicate undernutrition. These guidelines are approximate, and some patients may be misclassified as undernourished or obese because of individual variation.

**Body composition measures:** Used to estimate subcutaneous fat stores, muscle, and skeletal mass by measuring triceps skinfold thickness and mid-arm circumference. Validity depends on the accuracy of the measuring technique. This is not widely used in clinical settings because of limited practicality.

## Biochemical Data

**Visceral protein status:** Visceral protein levels are useful in assessing a patient's level of malnutrition and in evaluating the adequacy of nutritional therapy. Visceral protein levels measured may include serum albumin, transferrin, thyroxine-binding prealbumin, and retinol-binding protein (RBP). Albumin and transferrin have relatively long half-lives of 19 and 9 days, respectively, whereas prealbumin and RBP protein have short half-lives of 2 to 3 days and 12 hours, respectively. Albumin falls acutely in critical illness and is less useful as a marker of effectiveness of nutritional therapy in hospitalized patients, although it can be used as a baseline indicator of nutritional status and is useful as a prognostic indicator. Transferrin, because of its shorter half-life, is more useful than albumin in monitoring the adequacy of protein-energy intake. For evidence of the response to nutritional therapy, values for the short turnover proteins prealbumin and RBP are the most useful, although RBP is used less commonly in clinical settings. Many nonnutritional factors exist that result in altered levels of these protein parameters, and these should be taken into account when interpreting levels in regard to nutritional therapy. In states where inflammation is present, the value of these proteins as indicators of nutritional adequacy decreases. C-reactive protein is an indicator of the inflammatory process. An elevated C-reactive protein level indicates a shift from normal protein synthesis to acute-phase protein synthesis and may result in persistently low serum protein parameters despite appropriateness of nutritional therapy.

1. **Creatinine-height index:** Compares the patient's 24-hour urinary creatinine excretion with a predicted urinary creatinine excretion for individuals of the same height and gender as an evaluation of body muscle mass. Accuracy of results is affected by inadequate urine collection and the lack of age-referenced norms.

2. **Nitrogen balance:** A comparison of nitrogen (i.e., protein) intake with nitrogen excretion to determine adequacy of protein intake. A patient is in positive nitrogen balance if more nitrogen is consumed than is excreted and in negative nitrogen balance if less nitrogen is consumed than is excreted. Usually most nitrogen loss occurs through the urine, with a small amount lost via the skin and feces. Nitrogen balance studies require calculation of a 24-hour protein intake and a 24-hour urine collection. The usual goal in hospitalized patients is positive nitrogen balance (+2 to 4 g N if anabolism is desired), equal nitrogen balance, or decrease in the magnitude of nitrogen loss. Grams (g) of protein intake are multiplied by 16% to translate to grams of nitrogen, and the following equation is used:

$$\text{Nitrogen balance (g)} = \text{g protein intake } (0.16)$$
$$- (\text{g urinary urea nitrogen} + 4 \text{ g*})$$

*4 g is commonly used to account for nitrogen losses outside of urinary losses (i.e., feces and skin). Nonurea losses are greater if a patient has significant protein losses via draining wounds.

3. **Nutritional anemias:** Iron deficiency anemia results in red blood cells (RBCs) that are smaller than normal; that is, mean corpuscular volume (MCV) is less than normal, also known as microcytic. In addition, ferritin levels fall, plasma iron levels fall, and transferrin saturation decreases. However, other situations can affect these levels and should be considered for accurate diagnosis.

Folic acid or vitamin $B_{12}$ deficiency results in mega-loblastic anemia, characterized by large (macrocytic) immature RBCs that are larger than normal (increased MCV). Distinguishing folic acid deficiency from vitamin $B_{12}$ deficiency is determined with measuring serum $B_{12}$, serum folate and RBC folate levels. Nonnutritional anemias generally result in normocytic RBCs that have normal MCV.

4. **Other laboratory indices:** Include glucose, electrolytes, blood urea nitrogen (BUN), creatinine, complete blood counts, liver function tests, serum lipid levels, bleeding times, urine ketones, urine and serum osmolality, and arterial blood gases (ABG). These laboratory values help indicate tolerable levels or needed amounts of substrates, fluid, and electrolytes in nutritional support regimens and help dictate the aggressiveness with which nutrition support can be initiated.

## Estimating Energy Requirements

The primary goal of nutritional support is to meet energy requirements. Energy needs consist of basal needs for the body's metabolic processes, energy expended for activity, thermogenesis (energy expenditure to digest and metabolize food), energy required for growth, and additional energy requirements associated with illness, surgery, or trauma. With all the data collected, energy needs can be estimated with the following options:

1. **Indirect calorimetry:** Performed with a bedside metabolic cart by measuring oxygen consumption and carbon dioxide ($CO_2$) production, which are proportional to energy expenditure. This can be performed on independently breathing or ventilator-supported patients, if the ventilator settings can allow accurate testing. Results provide the most accurate measurement of energy expenditure and can help determine whether a patient's nutritional intake is appropriate. In addition, individual substrate (i.e., carbohydrate, fat, protein) utilization can be calculated.

2. **Harris-Benedict equations:** To determine basal energy expenditure (BEE), which is the energy expenditure of a healthy person just before or immediately on awakening before any activity occurs. The BEE accounts for 60% to

70% of the total daily energy expenditure.

BEE (males) = 66 + (13.8 × Weight in kg)
        + (5 × Height in cm) − (6.8 × age in years)

BEE (females) = 655 + (9.6 × Weight in kg)
        + (1.8 × Height in cm) − (4.7 × age in years)

BEE is then multiplied by appropriate factors to account for the patient's activity and condition. Commonly used factors are the following:

*Activity factor* = 1.2 for bedridden patients;

                1.3 for ambulatory patients

  *Injury factor* = 1.2 for minor surgery;

                1.35 for trauma; 1.6 for sepsis

BEE × activity factor × injury factor

    = total energy expenditure (TEE)

3. **Kilocalories/kilogram (kcal/kg):** A simple and quick method of estimating energy needs can be calculated at 25 to 35 kcal/kg for hospitalized adults, especially those who are at an appropriate body weight for their height. This method, because it does not take into account variables such as gender, age, stature, and severity of illness, is not as accurate as predictive equations or measurements that factor in these variables.

## Estimating Nutritional Requirements

1. **Distribution of calories:** Recommended percentages of total calories from carbohydrate, protein, and fat are approximately 50% to 55%, 15% to 20%, and 30%, respectively. The optimal percentages may be altered in various disease or inflammatory states.

   ■ *Carbohydrate requirements:* The preferred oxidative fuel of the body and the exclusive fuel for brain and nerve tissues. A minimum daily amount of carbohydrate of 50 to 100 g/day is necessary to avoid fat being excessively used for energy, in which case an accumulation of ketone bodies develops and acidosis results. If insufficient carbohydrate is consumed, the body can produce it by converting protein to glucose at the expense of body protein stores.

- *Protein requirements:* Usually 0.8 g protein/kg/day for healthy adults; increased to 1.5 to 2.5 g/kg/day in critically ill, hospitalized patients. Adequate carbohydrate must be provided or protein is used as an energy source and renders it unavailable for body protein synthesis.
- *Fat requirements:* Fat can be administered in minimal quantities to satisfy the need for essential fatty acids (equal to 2% to 4% of the energy requirement supplied by linoleic acid), or it can be offered in larger quantities (as tolerated) to meet energy needs.

2. **Vitamins, minerals, and electrolytes:** In general, the newest dietary reference intakes (DRI) help determine the optimal levels of intake of vitamins, minerals, and electrolytes. Some nutrients may need to be supplemented in increased amounts for certain disease states, therapies, or conditions to keep levels within the normal range.

3. **Fluid requirements:** Fluid requirements are estimated at 1 milliliter (mL)/kcal/day or 25 to 40 mL/kg weight per day. In addition to usual fluid needs, additional fluid is required for excessive urinary, fecal, blood, wound drainage, vomiting, or gastric decompression losses and with excessive insensible losses such as in febrile states.

## Nutritional Support Modalities

Two avenues of nutritional support exist: enteral and parenteral. Enteral nutrition is taken by mouth or is provided through a feeding tube or catheter that delivers nutrition distal to the oral cavity. Enteral nutrition is absorbed via the gastrointestinal (GI) tract. Parenteral nutrition (PN) is an intravenous (IV) solution infused through an IV line and does not rely on the GI tract for absorption. Cost, safety, and convenience have been the rationale for using enteral nutrition over PN support, but the physiologic benefits are a more compelling argument. Enteral nutrition stimulates accessory organs of digestion (i.e., pancreas, gallbladder, and biliary system) to function in their normal capacity and relies on hormonal controls to assist in appropriate digestion and absorption of nutrients. In addition, studies indicate that enteral feeding helps maintain gut mucosal integrity and prevent passage of bacteria across the GI tract into systemic circulation, thereby promoting intestinal health and reducing a potential source of infection.

## Enteral Nutrition

Wide varieties of formulas exist for provision of enteral nutrition that may be classified by several broad categories (Table 26-1).

The nutritional composition of enteral formulas may be broken down as follows:

1. **Carbohydrate:** Constitutes 30% to 90% of total calories. Most commercial enteral formulas are lactose-free because intolerance is common. The form of carbohydrate in enteral formulas ranges by the amount of hydrolysis from starch to monosaccharides.

2. **Fiber:** Included in many commercial formulas because of potential benefit in controlling blood glucose, reducing hyperlipidemia, and normalizing bowel function. May include a blend of insoluble and soluble fiber in the form of fiber from whole foods, soy fiber or polysaccharide, oat fiber, guar gum, pectin, or fructooligosaccharides. The infusion may need to be incorporated slowly to reduce transient symptoms of gas and abdominal distention if a low fiber diet/formula was previously used. Adequate fluid intake is important with fiber-containing enteral formulas.

3. **Protein:** Constitutes 6% to 25% of total calories. Provides a source of essential amino acids and nitrogen for protein synthesis. It is found in three forms in enteral formulas:
   - *Intact protein:* Protein found in its complete form that requires normal GI function for digestion and absorption.
   - *Hydrolyzed protein:* Protein that is broken down into smaller peptides to allow for easier digestion and absorption.
   - *Free amino acids:* Protein that requires no further digestion and is ready for absorption.

4. **Fat:** Provides 2% to 55% of total kcalories. Two forms are the primary sources:
   - *Long-chain triglycerides (LCTs):* Commonly vegetable oils that include linoleic acid as a source of essential fatty acids; facilitate the absorption of fat-soluble vitamins; some include omega-3 fatty acids from fish oils to lessen

Table 26-1  Types of enteral formulations

| Enteral Formula | Description |
|---|---|
| Intact nutrient or polymeric formulas | Require normal digestive and absorptive capability; consist of intact macronutrients; some may contain fiber; isotonic varieties provide 1 kcal/mL for normal fluid requirements and tolerance; concentrated, hypertonic formulas provide 1.5 to 2 kcal/mL for limited fluid tolerance; most are lactose-free; those intended for oral consumption have a higher sucrose content for enhanced palatability; some consist of blenderized whole foods |
| Predigested, elemental, semi-elemental, or chemically defined formulas | For limited digestive or absorptive capacity; macronutrients exist as maltodextrins, hydrolyzed cornstarch, oligosaccharides, disaccharides, or monosaccharides; low in long-chain fats or a high percentage of fat from MCT and completely or partially hydrolyzed protein to peptides or free amino acids; usually hypertonic |
| Disease-specific formulas | Polymeric formulas that are tailored to the nutritional needs of the particular disease state:<br><br>Diabetic formulas: Lower in carbohydrate (CHO); to help optimize glucose control usually isotonic<br><br>Pulmonary formulas: Higher in fat, lower in carbohydrates to help minimize $CO_2$ production if present; usually more concentrated (1.5 kcal/mL) to limit fluid provided |

*Continued*

Table 26-1 Types of enteral formulations—cont'd

| Enteral Formula | Description |
|---|---|
| | Renal formulas: Concentrated (2 kcal/mL) to limit fluid provided; level of protein differs depending on whether intended for patient on dialysis (higher protein content) or predialysis (lower protein content); electrolyte content is decreased or omitted; altered vitamin profile for renal disease; may contain higher percentage of protein as essential amino acids |
| | Hepatic formulas: Concentrated to limit fluid provided; low in sodium; higher percent of fat from MCT to contend with fat malabsorption; higher percentage of amino acids as branched-chain amino acids and smaller amounts of aromatic amino acids to improve nitrogen balance and lessen hepatic encephalopathy |
| Trauma formulas for metabolic stress or immune enhancement | Typically semielemental for ease in absorption; higher protein content; may contain any of combination of nutrients theorized to be beneficial in metabolic stress such as glutamine, arginine, nucleotides, branched-chain amino acids or omega-3 fatty acids |
| Modular products | Sources of additional protein; carbohydrate or fat that can be mixed into formulas to alter content when necessary; offer flexible tailoring of nutrients |

possible immune suppression connected with the metabolism of omega-6 fatty acids.

- *Medium-chain triglycerides (MCTs):* Made from coconut or palm kernel oil; able to be absorbed intact without normal pancreatic or hepatic function; not a source of essential amino acids; can be associated with nausea, vomiting, and diarrhea.

5. **Osmolality:** Osmolality is expressed as milliosmoles of solute per kilogram of solvent (mOsm/kg). The osmolality of normal body fluids is about 300 mOsm/kg. Solutions with an osmolality similar to that of normal body fluids are termed isotonic or isoosmolar. Solutions that have an osmolality greater than this are termed hyperosmolar or hypertonic and cause water to be drawn into those areas where the hyperosmolar solutions are. Hypertonic feedings may cause water to be drawn into the GI tract if given too rapidly, leading to cramping and diarrhea.

## Administration of Enteral Nutrition

The types of feeding tubes for enteral nutrition are usually classified by feeding route, size, or composition of material.

1. **Materials used:** Polyvinyl chloride (PVC), rubber, or latex tubes, although inexpensive, are not commonly used for long-term feeding. PVC becomes brittle and easily breakable with prolonged exposure to gastric acid. These tubes are also stiff, uncomfortable, and result in increased irritation. Long-term feeding tubes are usually made from polyurethane or silicone, which are softer, more comfortable, and longer lasting, although they have an increased risk of tube occlusion and tube walls may collapse with attempts at aspiration. Of these two, polyurethane tubes are stronger and have larger internal diameters that may help prevent tube clogging. Tubes occasionally used in surgical placement include Foley catheters, red rubber catheters, and T tubes.

2. **Size of tubes:** Outer diameter of tube lumen measured in French (F) units (No. 1 F = 0.33 mm). Larger tube diameters are necessary for fiber-containing or concentrated formulas and to allow administration by gravity without the use of a pump. Manufacturers provide information on the minimal French size of tubes necessary for individual product administration. The length of feeding tubes varies

by intended route of placement (gastric versus small bowel) and whether intended for infant, pediatric, or adult use.

3. **Gastric feeding tube:** Tube that is placed through the nares (nasogastric [NG] tube) or mouth (orogastric tube) into the stomach. This is usually intended for shorter term feeding (typically less than 6 to 8 weeks).

4. **Nasoenteric feeding tube:** Tube that is placed through the nares into the duodenum or jejunum. Some are larger tubes that have a second port to allow decompression of the stomach in concert with feeding into the small bowel. May allow for earlier enteral feeding after surgery because the small bowel is less affected than the stomach and colon by postoperative ileus. Also intended for short-term use.

5. **Gastrostomy tube (G-tube):** Tube that is inserted through the abdominal wall into the stomach. This may be placed surgically during an open laparotomy, endoscopically, radiologically, or laparoscopically. Endoscopically placed tubes are called percutaneous endoscopic gastrostomy (PEG) tubes, referring to the method of placement. G-tubes are usually larger in diameter (20 to 28° F) and more easily allow bolus or intermittent feeding by gravity. Intended for long-term use and indicated when trauma or obstruction prohibits access via the upper GI tract. "Low profile" G-tubes have the feeding connector close to the skin to allow for better concealment and to minimize pulling on the tube, although they require significant dexterity for formula administration.

6. **Jejunostomy tube (J-tube):** A tube that is inserted through the abdominal wall into the jejunum. This often is placed during an open surgical procedure because of technical difficulties with other methods, although it may be placed endoscopically (PEJ), radiologically, or laparoscopically. J-tubes require smaller tube diameters than G-tubes because of the diameter of the small bowel and therefore have a higher risk of tube occlusion. J-tubes are indicated when gastroparesis or gastric outlet obstruction/narrowing prohibits feeding into the stomach. Requires pump-facilitated continuous infusion to avoid dumping syndrome.

7. **Gastrostomy-jejunostomy tubes (G-J tubes):** A tube placed through the abdominal wall that has two ports and

lumens. One lumen ends in the stomach to allow for gastric decompression, and the other ends in the jejunum to allow for feeding. This type of tube is used when gastric suctioning is necessary because of gastroparesis or gastric outlet obstruction.

8. **Accessory items:** Y-ports, either built in as part of the system or added as a small adapter, allow concurrent administration of fluids or medications without disconnection of the feeding set. Some feeding pumps permit routine automatic administration of flush solutions as programmed into the machine by the nurse. Most enteral feeding connection sets are pump-specific and require the use of specific feeding bags or spike-sets.

For infusion rates, see Table 26-2. For collaborative management of complications, see Table 26-3.

## Parenteral Nutrition

Parenteral nutrition provides nutrition intravenously and does not use the GI tract for digestion or absorption of nutrients. Peripheral PN (PPN) is infused via a peripheral venous catheter (PVC), whereas total PN (TPN) is infused via a peripherally inserted central catheter (PICC) or central venous catheter (CVC). PN provides nutrition to patients who cannot receive enteral feedings or who are unable to digest or absorb sufficient nutrition via the GI tract because of obstruction, severe malabsorption, and ileus or bowel ischemia.

Parenteral solutions are composed of carbohydrate (dextrose), protein (amino acids), fat (lipids), electrolytes, vitamins, and trace elements. PN should be administered through a filter to prevent a precipitant from entering the bloodstream and forming an embolus.

1. **Carbohydrates:** Dextrose solutions are available in concentrations from 2.5% to 70% and provide energy, containing 3.4 calories/g of dextrose. Because of the administration of concentrated dextrose solutions, patients receiving PN should be monitored for glucose control until tolerance is established. Insulin may be added to PN solutions to treat hyperglycemia when present. Excessive carbohydrate administration may result in hepatic steatosis, hyperglycemia, or increased $CO_2$ production. Typical final concentrations

Table 26-2    Infusion rates

| Type | Typical Rate of Administration | Comments |
|------|-------------------------------|----------|
| **Bolus** (administer with syringe) | *Initiate:* 60-120 mL given 4-6 times per day. *Advancement:* Increase by 60 mL per bolus feeding to goal of 250-500 mL given 4-6 times per day. | Used for gastric feedings; useful in home setting or in extended care facilities; mimics normal eating schedule of divided meals throughout day; allows more freedom for ambulation and activity; may cause nausea, cramping, diarrhea, or reflux. |
| **Intermittent** (administer by gravity with feeding container and gravity set) | *Initiate:* 120 mL administered over 20- to 30-minute periods throughout day. *Advancement:* Increase formula by 60 mL each feeding as tolerated until goal reached. | Used for gastric feedings; should not exceed 30 mL/minute; less likely to cause GI intolerance than bolus feedings because of slower administration. |

in TPN solutions may range from 15% to 35% in more concentrated solutions. Final concentrations in PPN solutions are usually 5% to 10%.

2. **Protein:** Synthetic crystalline amino acid solutions provide essential amino acids and nitrogen for protein synthesis. Special amino acid formulations for specific circumstances (e.g., stress, liver, or renal disease or for pediatric populations) are available. Commercial amino acid solutions are available in concentrations of 3.5% to 20% with typical final concentrations in TPN solutions ranging from

Table 26-2   Infusion rates—cont'd

| Type | Typical Rate of Administration | Comments |
|---|---|---|
| **Continuous** (administer with infusion pump) | *Initiate:* Isotonic formulas at 30-50 mL/hour; hypertonic formulas at 15-25 mL/hour; infuse over 12-24 hours per day.<br><br>*Advancement:* Increase by 25 mL every 8 hours as tolerated until goal rate reached. | May be used for any type of feeding tube; required for small bowel because small bowel cannot act as reservoir for large volumes of formula within short instillation time; usually most easily tolerated feeding method and therefore usually method used in critically ill patients or used for initiation of feedings until tolerance is determined; incurs additional expense for infusion pump and supplies compared with bolus feedings. |

4% to 9% and in PPN solutions usually less than 3%. Amino acid solutions may provide some electrolyte content, depending on the formulation used.

3. **Fat:** IV lipid emulsions of soybean or safflower oil with egg yolk phospholipids are isotonic and available in concentrations from 10% to 30%. They provide a source of concentrated calories and essential fatty acids. When infused separately from the PN solution, 10% to 20% solutions are used and the infusion time for a single bottle is limited to 12 hours to avoid microbial contamination. Adverse reactions to lipid emulsions may occur, and the initial

Table 26-3 Collaborative management of complications in tube-fed patients

| Complications | Suggested Management Strategy |
|---|---|
| Nausea and vomiting<br>Reflux<br>High gastric residuals<br>Aspiration | Decrease rate or feeding volume until tolerance is achieved before increasing further; hold feedings for 1 hour if high (> 150 mL) residual volumes of formula until residual has decreased; consider changing to continuous feedings; consider gastric motility agents; consider changing to lower fat, fiber-free, or isotonic formula; ensure head of bed is elevated at least 30 degrees while feeding; consider postpyloric feedings |
| Pneumothorax<br>Aspiration | Obtain radiograph confirmation of placement of NG/nasoenteric feeding tubes before initial use or when tube migration is suspected; stop tube advancement during placement if resistance is encountered; monitor for respiratory distress (coughing, shortness of breath, inability to speak) |
| Product odor/taste | Mask with flavoring; provide regular mouth care |
| Blocked tube | Prevention is key: flush tube with 30 mL water before and after checking residuals and before and after administering bolus or intermittent feedings; flush with 30 mL water every 4-6 hours during continuous feedings; ensure adequate tube size for concentrated or fiber-containing formulas; do not combine medications or mix with formula because incompatibilities exist and may cause clumping of formula; flush after each medication instillation; substitute liquid medication preparations where possible or crush to fine powder before administering |

infusion rate of lipids should be no faster than 1 mL/minute for the first 15 to 30 minutes until tolerance is established.

4. **Total nutrient admixtures (TNAs):** Also called 3-in-1 admixtures, these solutions combine dextrose, amino acids, and lipids in one container as opposed to a 2-in-1 admixture that provides dextrose and amino acids in one container with the lipid emulsion provided separately. TNAs may ease administration, lessen manipulation of the system, and reduce necessary supplies (e.g., pumps and IV tubing) but are less stable and increase difficulty in visualizing particulate matter or precipitates in the solution. In addition, a larger filter of 1.2 μ is used with TNAs to allow the larger lipid molecules to pass, instead of the smaller 0.22-μ filter used with the 2-in-1 admixture, which can eliminate smaller precipitates or contaminants.

## Administration of Parenteral Nutrition

In selection of an administration site, the following should be considered:

1. **CVC or PICC:** Central catheters whose distal tip lies in the superior or inferior vena cava where the volume of blood flow rapidly dilutes the hypertonic solutions and decreases the irritation of vein walls. In adults, common placement is via the subclavian, jugular, or femoral veins. A physician performs placement (with the exception that nurses can be certified to place PICC lines). Used to administer TPN.

2. **PVC:** An IV placed into a peripheral vein, usually of the forearm or hand. Because of limited vein tolerance, PPN solutions must not exceed an osmolarity of 900 mOsm/L and thus are more dilute and require increased volumes to deliver significant amounts of calories and protein. Lipid emulsions are well tolerated peripherally because of the isotonicity of the solution and can help to provide concentrated calories with PPN. PPN given via a PVC is best suited for individuals with lower nutritional requirements and more liberal fluid tolerance who do not require PN for an extended period and for those for whom CVC access is unavailable.

PN is administered with an infusion pump at a consistent rate that may typically be 50 to 100 mL/hour. It may need to be initiated at a lower rate and advanced slowly depending on a patient's status and tolerance. Central catheter site care requires meticulous attention because catheters allow easy entrance for microorganisms into a major vein, which places the patient at high risk for infection.

For types of catheters, see Table 26-4. For the management of complications, see Table 26-5.

## Transitional Feeding

A period of adjustment may be needed before discontinuing nutrition support. Enteral formulas and oral supplements should be tapered as oral intake of food increases. Tube feeding regimens may be changed to a nocturnal infusion as diet intake increases to optimize appetite for meals. Patients receiving PN may have some bowel atrophy and may need time for adjustment before the bowel can fully resume usual functioning. Tapering of PN can begin as enteral feedings provide increasing proportions of requirements.

## Potential Fluid, Electrolyte, and Acid-Base Disturbances in Enteral and Parenteral Nutrition

1. **Refeeding syndrome:** A situation requiring particular consideration when providing nutritional support to severely malnourished patients. Patients who sustain a prolonged period of starvation have resulting lower total body levels of circulating phosphorus, magnesium, and potassium. When these patients suddenly have adequate energy intake (as can occur with enteral nutrition or PN especially), an increased insulin response results in an intracellular shift of these electrolytes with the potential for severely depleted serum levels. In addition, abnormal glucose levels and congestive heart failure may be seen. Resulting organ dysfunction may be severe enough to be fatal. Prevention of refeeding syndrome involves initiating feedings at a lower calorie level and increasing to goal slowly over a period of days and anticipating increased electrolyte requirements with frequent monitoring and supplementation of phosphorus, potassium, and magnesium as needed. Refeeding syndrome can occur in patients on oral diets as well, particularly in patients who have the appetite and

Table 26-4   Parenteral access

| Catheter | Description |
|---|---|
| **Short-Term Central Access** | |
| Percutaneous nontunneled catheters | May be inserted at bedside with only local anesthetic. Inserted via subclavian, jugular, or femoral vein. In lines with multiple lumens, dedication of one lumen for TPN is common (usually most distal port), enabling other lumens to be used for medication administration, other IV fluids, and blood aspiration. Can be used for several weeks if line infection avoided. Offer easy removal and ability to exchange catheters over guidewire. |
| **Long-Term Central Access** | |
| Tunneled catheter (e.g., Hickman) | Placed in operating room with general anesthesia. Subcutaneous tunnel is created so that catheter exits skin several inches away from its venous entry site (cephalic, subclavian, or internal jugular vein) to hinder microbial entry into vein. Can be used for years. |
| Implanted port | Placed in operating room with general anesthesia. Catheter is located completely subcutaneously, with disk that can be palpated and accessed with a special 90-degree needle for use. Site care is required only when accessed. Requires surgical procedure for removal. Ideal for intermittent or infrequent IV therapies. |

NOTE: Peripheral devices cannot be used for central line TPN administration but only for solutions intended for peripheral use (PPN).

*Continued*

Table 26-4  Parenteral access—cont'd

| Catheter | Description |
| --- | --- |
| PICC | Catheter is inserted into antecubital vein and then threaded via subclavian vein to superior vena cava (SVC). Can be inserted at bedside by specially trained nurses. May provide less risk of complications than other central lines. |
| **Peripheral Device** | |
| Single/dual lumen | Short-term (few day) use. Least risk for catheter-related infections. |
| Midline catheters | Inserted 5 to 7 inches into vein with catheter tip terminating in proximal portion of upper extremity. Can be used for 2 to 4 weeks. |
| Midclavicular catheters | Catheters with tip located in proximal axillary or subclavian veins. May be used for 2 to 3 months. |

ability to consume adequate oral intake but because of social or physical limitations were unable to consume adequate intake before admission (e.g., homeless or neglected individuals).

2. **Hypervolemia:** May be a result of excessive fluid volume provided by the PN or enteral nutrition solution or the volume of supplementary water. May also be seen in renal dysfunction, congestive heart failure, or hepatic failure. Refeeding a malnourished individual results in raised insulin levels that decrease excretion of sodium and water by the kidneys. The retention of sodium and water is called refeeding edema (see Chapter 6).

3. **Hypovolemia:** May have intravascular volume depletion from hypoalbuminemia resulting in decreased oncotic

Table 26-5   Management of complications in patients
receiving parenteral nutrition

| Potential Complications | Management Strategy |
| --- | --- |
| Pneumothorax | Obtain radiograph immediately after insertion to determine placement and to monitor for pneumothorax before using. Observe for diminished or unequal breath sounds, tachycardia, dyspnea, and labored breathing. |
| Arterial injury | Observe for pulsatile, bright red blood return into syringe. Assist healthcare provider with immediate removal of needle and apply pressure for 10 minutes anteriorly and posteriorly at point of penetration. |
| Catheter occlusion | Ensure routine line flushing. If solution is infusing sluggishly, check to see if line is kinked or pinched and flush line with normal saline. If line is occluded, try to aspirate clot and contact healthcare provider, who may prescribe thrombolytic agent. |
| Hypoglycemia/ hyperglycemia | Administer 10% dextrose in peripheral vein at same rate as TPN solution if catheter becomes dysfunctional or TPN is abruptly stopped and monitor glucose levels every 1 hour until stable. Rapid increases or decreases in rate should be avoided. Perform fingerstick glucose checks every 4-6 hours or as needed until stable to monitor for hyperglycemia. |

*Continued*

Table 26-5   Management of complications in patients receiving parenteral nutrition—cont'd

| Potential Complications | Management Strategy |
| --- | --- |
| Catheter-related infection | Ensure that sterile technique is used for catheter insertion and dressing changes and aseptic technique is used for tubing changes. Ensure routine dressing changes and site care. Hang single solution of PN no longer than 24 hours; hang bottle of lipid emulsion no longer than 12 hours; use 0.22-$\mu$ filter with PN solutions. |

pressure and increased fluid loss into tissue, known as "third-spacing" of fluid. Can occur with excessive diuresis or inadequate fluid provision in the nutrition support regimen. May be seen in patients with excessive fluid losses from vomiting, diarrhea, bleeding, and wound drainage or with increased insensible losses from fever or diaphoresis.

4. **Hypernatremia:** Seen with inadequate fluid administration or excessive fluid losses. May be the result of excessive sodium intake. All patients should be carefully monitored for sodium intake from medications, blood products, and feedings. Water intake should be carefully monitored to ensure the patient is receiving adequate fluid (see Chapter 7).

5. **Hyponatremia:** Stable patients on long-term enteral feeding regimens, most of which contain limited sodium, may experience hyponatremia (see Chapter 7). May also be seen with excessive fluid administration or dilutional states seen in conjunction with congestive heart failure, renal or hepatic failure, or syndrome of inappropriate antidiuretic hormone (SIADH).

6. **Hyperkalemia:** May occur with excessive enteral or parenteral potassium supplementation. May result from metabolic acidosis in which potassium ions are exchanged extracellularly for hydrogen ions to help lessen acidosis.

May also occur in renal insufficiency (see Chapter 8) and with cell lysis. May occur with the use of potassium-sparing diuretics.

7. **Hypokalemia:** May occur with refeeding syndrome and with inadequate potassium provision. Metabolic alkalosis may result in hypokalemia as potassium is moved intracellularly in exchange for hydrogen ions. Excessive diarrhea or fistula losses and certain medications (e.g., potassium-losing diuretics and amphotericen B) result in excessive potassium losses.

8. **Hyperphosphatemia:** Usually occurs in renal insufficiency. May be seen with excessive phosphorus supplementation.

9. **Hypophosphatemia:** Occurs in the refeeding of a malnourished patient. Common in alcoholism. May occur with prolonged use of phosphate-binding antacids. May result from insulin therapy. Seen with inadequate phosphorus administration.

10. **Hypermagnesemia:** May be seen in renal insufficiency or with excessive magnesium provision or use of magnesium-containing laxatives.

11. **Hypomagnesemia:** Low levels occur in patients with severe malnutrition during rapid refeeding. Also seen with excessive GI losses and with insulin or amphotericin B administration. May occur with inadequate magnesium provision.

12. **Hyperglycemia:** Anticipated in patients with diabetes and those receiving steroids but may also occur in otherwise normoglycemic patients on TPN as a result of the concentration of dextrose. May be seen in sepsis or postoperative stress. Seen in chromium deficiency and excessive carbohydrate intake.

13. **Hypoglycemia:** May occur if abrupt cessation of the TPN occurs, as with sudden line removal or dysfunction or with cycling of TPN. May be seen with excessive insulin administration or with cessation of enteral nutrition after scheduled insulin has been administered.

14. **Acid-base disturbances:** May be seen because of excessive intake of acetate via the PN solution or overfeeding (especially of carbohydrates) leading to increased $CO_2$ production.

## Nursing Diagnoses and Interventions

**Imbalanced nutrition: less than body requirements** related to inability to ingest, digest, or absorb nutrients.

**Desired outcome:** Within 7 days of initiating PN or enteral nutrition, the patient has adequate nutrition as evidenced by appropriate weight gain or cessation of weight loss; improved or normal measures of visceral protein stores or other laboratory indices; a state of nitrogen balance or lessened nitrogen loss; the presence of wound granulation; and an absence of or improving infection.

*For oral nutrition:*

1. Ensure timely nutritional screening and assessment of the patient with appropriate documentation and reassessment. Make a referral to a dietitian if indicated.
2. Position the patient in a high Fowler's position for eating and assist with feeding or setting up the meal for eating as needed. Involve significant others at mealtimes for companionship and encouragement. Provide small frequent feedings of a diet compatible with the disease state and the patient's ability to ingest foods.
3. Respect the patient's food aversions and try to maximize food preferences.
4. Provide liquid nutritional supplements as prescribed. Serve them cold or over ice to enhance palatability.
5. Document intake; use daily calorie counts as ordered or indicated.
6. Weigh weekly or more frequently if indicated.
7. Provide psychological support and encouragement.

*For enteral nutrition and PN:*

1. Ensure timely nutritional screening and assessment of the patient with appropriate documentation and reassessment. Make referral to nutrition support personnel if indicated.
2. Administer formula at the prescribed rate or volume. Check the infused volume and rate hourly.
3. Monitor laboratory data daily: blood glucose, BUN, creatinine, and electrolytes may be ordered daily. Visceral protein parameters, blood lipid levels, CBC, bleeding times, and liver function tests may be monitored weekly. Document and evaluate the findings.

4. Record intake and output (I&O) carefully, tracking fluid balance trends.
5. Weigh the patient twice weekly or as ordered; consistently document findings.
6. Document TPN, lipids, or tube feeding (TF) intake volume and any intolerances to the prescribed regimen.
7. Discuss intolerances with healthcare provider as needed.

**Risk for aspiration** related to GI feeding, site of feeding tube, delayed gastric emptying, or absence of normal protective mechanisms.

**Desired outcome:** Patient is free of aspiration problems as evidenced by auscultation of clear lung sounds, vital signs (VS) within the patient's normal limits, and an absence of signs of respiratory distress.

1. Verify feeding tube position with all available methods, including confirming the tube position with a radiograph after initial placement and with suspected displacement, auscultating for whoosh of air in stomach when air is instilled in feeding tube with a syringe, and possibly monitoring pH of feeding tube aspirate. Gently aspirate a small-bore tube; it may collapse with the pressure of aspiration.
2. Mark the tube or note tube markings to determine tube migration and secure the tubing in place; reassess placement every 4 hours or before each feeding.
3. Assess respiratory status every 4 hours for unexplained pulmonary infiltrates, noting the respiratory rate and effort and adventitious breath sounds.
4. Monitor VS every 4 hours; promptly report a fever of unexplained origin.
5. Auscultate bowel sounds, percuss abdomen, and assess abdominal contour and girth every 8 hours. Consult the healthcare provider if bowel sounds are absent or high pitched, the abdomen becomes distended, gastric residuals are higher than the tolerable threshold (commonly 150 to 200 mL), the patient has nausea, or vomiting occurs. Replace removed residual unless vomiting occurs.
6. Elevate the head of the bed greater than 30 degrees during feeding and 1 hour after feeding. If this is not possible for the patient, turn the patient to a slightly elevated right

side-lying position to enhance gravity flow from the greater stomach curvature to the pylorus.

7. Delay the next feeding for 1 hour and recheck the residual. Resume feeding if residual is less than 150 to 200 mL or the prescribed threshold. Stop tube feeding ½ to 1 hour before physical therapy for the chest, suctioning, or supine placement of the patient if anticipated.

8. Discuss with the healthcare provider the possibility of advancing the feeding tube postpylorically if the risk of aspiration is high because of gastroparesis.

9. As prescribed, administer metoclopramide or erythromycin to promote gastric motility and emptying.

10. If your institution has the protocol in place, test pulmonary secretions for glucose, which may indicate the aspiration of formula (is falsely positive when blood is in the sample).

11. Keep the endotracheal/tracheostomy cuff inflated during feeding.

**Constipation (or risk for)** related to inadequate fluid and fiber in the diet.

**Desired outcome:** The patient has a soft bowel movement within 2 to 3 days of the diagnosis (or within the patients' usual pattern).

1. Assess the intake of free water. Normally, water intake should be 1 mL/kcal of formula or 25 to 40 mL/kg of body weight (may need to use adjusted body weight for obesity).

2. Give free water every 4 hours or as prescribed. Use of feeding pumps that allow automatic administration of free water at programmed intervals may help ensure adequate free water intake.

3. Recommend a change of formula to one that has fiber added if adequate fluid can be tolerated (not recommended if fluid restriction is necessary because of the potential for hard impacted stools).

4. Use of laxatives as prescribed.

5. Monitor for impaction.

6. Encourage physical activity as tolerated.

**Diarrhea (or risk for)** related to tube feeding, lactose intolerance, bacterial contamination, osmolality intolerance, medications, or a low fiber content.

**Desired outcome:** The patient has formed stools within 2 to 3 days of intervention.

1. Assess the abdomen and GI status by monitoring bowel sounds, distention, cramping, and consistency and frequency of bowel movements; monitor skin turgor, urine output, urine specific gravity, and other indications of hydration if diarrhea is present.

2. Monitor I&O balance carefully.

3. Bolus feedings may need to be changed to intermittent or continuous feeding methods if diarrhea occurs.

4. In cases of lactose intolerance, ensure use of a lactose-free product.

5. For bacterial contamination:
   - Obtain a stool specimen for culture and sensitivity; check for *Clostridium difficile*.
   - Use aseptic technique in handling the feeding tube, enteral formulas, and feeding sets or syringes.
   - Change feeding sets every 24 hours.
   - Refrigerate all opened products; date and time when opened and discard after 48 hours of opening.
   - With an open system in which formula is poured into a feeding bag, only add enough formula that can be infused within 8 hours and discard formula hanging for more than 8 hours. With a closed system in which the feeding container is spiked with a feeding set, hang formula for 24 hours and discard remainder after 24 hours.

6. For osmolality intolerance, determine the osmolality of the feeding formula (this is listed on the container or may be obtained from the dietitian or pharmacist). Isotonic formulas have an osmolality of about 300 mOsm/kg. If a hypertonic formula is used, the infusion rate or volume may need to be reduced temporarily. If diarrhea continues, consider changing to an isotonic formula.

7. Medications:
   - Monitor the use of antibiotics, antacids, antidysrhythmics, aminophylline, cimetidine, and electrolyte supplementation and the use of sorbitol in liquid medications that may contribute to diarrhea. Enlist the help of a pharmacist as needed.

- Use antidiarrheal agents as prescribed to decrease GI motility (if *Clostridium difficile* has been ruled out) if frequent episodes of diarrhea occur.
- Use antidiarrheal agents that absorb water or add bulk if stools are watery but not frequent.

8. Consider a fiber-containing TF formula or add bulk-forming agents to the regimen as prescribed.
9. Monitor serum albumin levels; low serum albumin levels may contribute to bowel edema and intestinal malabsorption. The regimen may need to be altered to contend with malabsorption.
10. Use an infusion pump when feeding into the small bowel.

**Impaired swallowing (or risk for)** related to decreased or absent gag reflex, facial paralysis, mechanical obstruction, fatigue, and decreased strength of muscles involved in mastication.

**Desired outcome:** Before foods or fluids are initiated, the patient demonstrates adequate cough and gag reflexes and the ability to ingest food via the phases of swallowing as instructed.

1. Assess oral motor function within 72 hours of the patient's admission or on progression to an oral diet.
2. Assess cough and gag reflexes before the first feeding. Initially liquids and solids may be difficult for the patient to manage. Offer semisolid foods and progress to a thicker texture as tolerated. Assist the patient throughout the phases of ingesting food: opening the mouth, inserting food, closing the lips, chewing, transferring food from side to side in the mouth and then to the back of the oral cavity, elevating the tongue to the roof of the mouth, and swallowing between breaths.
3. Order extra sauces, gravies, or liquids if dryness of the oral cavity impairs the patient's swallowing ability. Suggest that the patient moisten each bite of food with these substances.
4. If tolerated, keep the patient in a high Fowler's position for 30 minutes after eating to minimize the risk of aspiration.
5. Provide mouth care before and after meals and dietary supplements as needed.
6. Provide small frequent meals; six feedings per day may be better tolerated than three feedings.

7. Provide foods at temperatures acceptable to the patient.
8. Respect food aversions and honor food preferences whenever possible.
9. Provide oral supplements or tube feeding supplementation as prescribed. Advise the patient of the transition status and praise the patient's progress.
10. In conjunction with a speech, physical, or occupational therapist, assist in retraining or facilitating the patient's swallowing.
11. Monitor and record the patient's intake (via calorie count if ordered) and output.

**Impaired tissue integrity (or risk for)** related to mechanical irritant (presence of feeding tube).

**Desired outcome:** The patient's tissue is intact, with an absence of: erosion around orifices, excoriation, skin rash, mucous membrane breakdown, and ulcers.

*For nasoenteric tube:*

1. Assess the skin for irritation or tenderness every 8 hours.
2. Use the smallest bore tube possible.
3. If long-term support is needed, discuss the potential for a G-tube or J-tube with the healthcare provider.
4. Apply petroleum ointment to the patient's lips every 2 hours.
5. Have the patient brush the teeth and tongue twice a day if possible.
6. Apply water-soluble lubricant to the nares prn.
7. Alter the position of the tube as needed to avoid pressure on underlying tissue. Use hypoallergenic tape to anchor the tube.

*For G-J tube:*

1. Assess the site for erythema, drainage, tenderness, and odor every 4 hours.
2. Secure the tube in a way that avoids tension on the patient's tissue and skin.
3. For new sites, cleanse the skin with half-strength hydrogen peroxide solution. Dress with split $4 \times 4$s and tape with paper or hypoallergenic tape.
4. For healed sites, cleanse the skin with soap and water and pat dry daily.
5. If necessary, dress the site with split $4 \times 4$s and tape with paper or hypoallergenic tape.

**Risk for infection** related to invasive procedures, malnutrition, or a suppressed immune system.

**Desired outcome:** The patient is free of infection as evidenced by temperature and VS within normal limits, a white blood cell (WBC) count within normal limits, and the absence of clinical signs of sepsis (e.g., erythema and swelling at catheter insertion site, chills, fever, glucose intolerance).

1. Ensure adequate nutritional support based on the individual's needs; reassess weekly.
2. Monitor laboratory parameters indicative of infection (WBC count and differential, glucose).
3. Check blood glucose via fingerstick every 6 hours for elevated values if indicated.
4. Examine catheter insertion sites every 8 hours for erythema, swelling, tenderness, or purulent discharge.
5. Use meticulous sterile technique when changing central line dressing, containers, or lines. Use sterile gloves and masks per agency policy. Do not use a central line lumen that is infusing PN to draw blood, monitor pressure, or administer medications or other fluids if possible to minimize contamination.
6. Change all administration sets within the time frame established by the institution.
7. Do not hang a single TPN solution for greater than 24 hours or a bottle of lipid emulsion for greater than 12 hours.

**Ineffective cardiopulmonary tissue perfusion (or risk for)** related to interruption of arterial flow (air embolus).

**Desired outcome:** Patient has adequate cardiopulmonary tissue perfusion as evidenced by VS, ABG values, and oximetry readings within the patient's normal limits and the absence of tachypnea, cyanosis, chest pain, tachycardia, heart murmur, and hypotension.

1. Administer only IV fluid intended for peripheral venous access until the chest radiograph verifies proper central access position.
2. Position the patient in the Trendelenburg position when changing tubing or when neck vein catheters are inserted or removed.
3. If possible, teach the patient Valsalva's maneuver for use during tubing changes or apply abdominal pressure.
4. Use Luer-Lok connectors on all connections and change routinely.

5. Tape all tubing connections longitudinally to prevent disconnection.

6. Monitor the patient for chest pain, tachycardia, tachypnea, cyanosis, and hypotension. If air embolus is suspected, listen for crackles and $S_3$ and $S_4$ gallop rhythms.

7. If air embolus is suspected, clamp the catheter and turn the patient to a left side-lying Trendelenburg position to trap air in the right ventricle. Give oxygen and monitor VS. Notify the physician immediately.

8. Use an occlusive dressing over the insertion site for 24 hours after the catheter is removed to prevent air entry via catheter-sinus tract.

**Deficient fluid volume (or risk for)** related to failure of regulatory mechanisms, hyperglycemia, and hyperosmolar hyperglycemic nonketotic syndrome (HHNS).

**Desired outcome:** The patient's hydration status is adequate, as evidenced by baseline VS, serum glucose less than 200 mg/dL, balanced I&O, urine specific gravity of 1.01 to 1.025, and serum electrolytes within normal limits.

1. Assess the rate and volume of nutritional support hourly. Reset to the prescribed rate as indicated. To minimize the risk of HHNS, increase the rate slowly until glucose control is established.

2. Weigh the patient daily; monitor I&O carefully.

3. Consult with the healthcare provider regarding a decreased urine output.

4. Check urine specific gravity as ordered; consult with the healthcare provider regarding a value greater than 1.035.

5. Monitor serum osmolality and electrolytes daily or as indicated; notify the healthcare provider of abnormalities.

6. Monitor for circulatory overload during fluid replacement, adventitious lung sounds (especially crackles/rales), peripheral edema, and jugular distention.

7. Monitor for hyperglycemia. Perform a fingerstick glucose check every 4 to 6 hours or as needed until stable. Administer insulin (commonly a sliding scale) as prescribed to keep blood glucose levels within the desirable range or less than 200 mg/dL.

8. Provide 1 mL of free water for each calorie of enteral formula (or 25 to 40 mL/kg of body weight).

# Selected
# References

Abelow B: *Understanding acid-base,* Baltimore, 1998, Williams & Wilkins.

Adrogue HJ, Madias NE: Hypernatremia, *N Engl J Med* 342(20): 1493-1499, 2000.

Adrogue HJ, Madias NE: Management of life threatening acid-base disorders, *N Engl J Med* 338(1):26-34, 1998.

Adrogue HJ, Madias NE: Management of life threatening acid-base disorders, *N Engl J Med* 338(2):107-111, 1998.

Adrogue HE, Adrogue HJ: Acid base physiology, *Respir Care* 46(4):328-341, 2001.

Ahmed J, Weisberg LS: Hyperkalemia in dialysis patients, *Semin Dial* 14(5):348-356, 2001.

Al-Saden P: Hepatic failure. In Swearingen PL, Keen JH, editors: *Manual of critical care nursing: nursing interventions and collaborative management,* ed 4, St Louis, 2001, Mosby.

American Society for Parenteral and Enteral Nutrition: *The A.S.P.E.N. nutrition support practice manual,* Silver Spring, Md, 1998, American Society for Parenteral and Enteral Nutrition.

Ammon S: Managing patients with heart failure, *AJN* 101(12):34-40, 2001.

Ayus JC, Arieff AI: Chronic hyponatremic encephalopathy in postmenopausal women: association of therapies with morbidity and mortality, *JAMA* 281(24):2299-2304, 1999.

Bagley SM: Nutritional needs of the acutely ill with acute wounds, *Crit Care Nurs Clin North Am* 8(2):159-167, 1996.

Baird MS: Congestive heart failure/pulmonary edema. In Swearingen PL, Keen JH, editors: *Manual of critical care nursing: nursing interventions and collaborative management,* ed 4, St Louis, 2001, Mosby.

Beck LH: The aging kidney: defending a delicate balance of fluid and electrolytes, *Geriatrics* 55(4):26-32, 2000.

Berry BE, Pinard AE: Assessing tissue oxygenation, *Crit Care Nurse* 22(3):22-42, 2002.

Balas MC: Prone positioning of patients with acute respiratory distress syndrome: applying research to practice, *Crit Care Nurs* 20(1):24-36, 2000.

Blanning A, Westfall JM, Shaughnessy AF: How soon should serum potassium levels be monitored for patients started on diuretics? *J Fam Pract* 50(3):207-208, 2001.

Block GA: Control of serum phosphorus: implications for coronary artery calcification and calcific uremic arteriolopathy (calciphylaxis), *Curr Opin Nephrol Hypertens* 10(6):741-747, 2001.

Bohn D: Problems associated with intravenous fluid administration in children: do we have the right solutions? *Curr Opin Pediatr* 12(3):217-221, 2000.

Brater DC: Pharmacology of diuretics, *Am J Med Sci* 319(1):38-50, 2000.

Braxmeyer DL, Keyes JL: The pathophysiology of potassium balance, *Crit Care Nurs* 16(5):59-71, 1996.

Bugg NC, Jones JA: Hypophosphatemia: pathophysiology, effects and management on the intensive care unit, *Anaesthesia* 53(9):895-902, 1998.

Burchell SA, Ho HC, Yu M et al: Effects of methamphetamine on trauma patients: a cause of severe metabolic acidosis? *Crit Care Med* 28(6):2112-2115, 2000.

Bushinsky DA, Monk RD: Calcium, *Lancet* 352(9124):306-311, 1998.

Braunwald E, Fauci AS, Kasper DL et al, editors: *Harrison's principles of internal medicine*, ed 15, New York, 2001, McGraw Hill.

Campbell D: How acute renal failure puts the brakes on kidney function, *Nursing 2003* 33(1):59-62, 2003.

Carelock J, Clark AP: Heart failure: pathophysiologic mechanisms, *AJN* 101(12):26-33, 2001.

Carlson RW, Keshavamurth L: Fluid and electrolyte emergencies: some signposts to safe management, *J Crit Illn* 14(10):554-562, 1999.

Cohn JN, Kowey PR, Whelton PK et al: New guidelines for potassium replacement in clinical practice: a contemporary review by the National Council on Potassium in Clinical Practice, *Arch Intern Med* 160(16):2429-2436, 2000.

Dahan E, Orbach S, Weiss YG: Fluid management in trauma, *Int Anesthesiol Clin* 38(4):141-148, 2000.

Deftos LJ: Hypercalcemia: mechanisms, differential diagnosis, and remedies, *Postgrad Med* 100(6):119-126, 1996.

DePriest J: Reversing oliguria in critically ill patients, *Postgrad Med* 102(3):245-263, 1997.

Duerksen DR, Papineau N, Siemens J et al: Peripherally inserted enteral catheters for parenteral nutrition: a comparison with centrally inserted catheters, *J Parenter Enteral Nutr* 23(2):85-89, 1999.

Dunn A, Chow MS, Kluger J: A natriuretic peptide with hemodynamic benefits in patients with acute decompensated CHF, *Formulary* 34:123-131, 1999.

*Drug facts and comparisons,* St Louis, 2003, Wolters Kluwer.

Dubose T, Hamm L, editors: *Acid-base and electrolyte disorders: a companion to Brenner & Rector's The Kidney,* Philadelphia, 2003, WB Saunders.

Evans-Stoner N: Nutritional assessment: a practical approach, *Nurs Clin North Am* 32(4):637-650, 1997.

Epstein SK, Singh N: Respiratory acidosis, *Respir Care* 46(4):366-383, 2001.

Fabian B: Intravenous complication: infiltration, *J Intraven Nurs* 23(4):229-231, 2000.

Farthing MJ: Oral rehydration: an evolving solution, *J Pediatr Gastroenterol Nutr* 34(suppl 1):S64-S67, 2002.

Fencl V et al: Diagnosis of metabolic acid-base disturbances in critically ill patients, *Am J Respir Crit Care Med* 162:2246-2251, 2000.

Foster GT, Vaziri ND, Sassoon CS: Respiratory alkalosis, *Respir Care* 46(4):384-391, 2001.

Fraser CL, Arieff AI: Epidemiology, pathophysiology, and management of hyponatremic encephalopathy, *Am J Med* 102(1):67-77, 1997.

Fried LF, Palevsky PM: Hyponatremia and hypernatremia, *Med Clin North Am* 81(3):585-609, 1997.

Gay-George B: Acute pancreatitis. In Swearingen PL, Keen JH, editors: *Manual of critical care nursing: nursing interventions and collaborative management,* ed 4, St Louis, 2001, Mosby.

Gennari FJ: Current concepts—hypokalemia, *N Engl J Med* 339(7): 451-458, 1998.

Goll C: Respiratory dysfunctions. In Swearingen PL, Keen JH, editors: *Manual of critical care nursing: nursing interventions and collaborative management,* ed 4, St Louis, 2001, Mosby.

Gottschlich MM, editor: The science and practice of nutrition support: a case-based core curriculum, Silver Spring, Md, 2001, American Society for Parenteral and Enteral Nutrition.

Greenberg A: Hyperkalemia—treatment options, *Semin Nephrol* 18(1):46-57, 1998.

Greenberg A: Diuretic complications, *Am J Med Sci* 319(1):10-24, 2000.

Gunn V, Nechyba C, editors: *The Harriet Lane handbook,* ed 16, St Louis, 2002, Mosby.

Halperin ML, Goldstein MB: *Fluid, electrolyte and acid-base physiology,* ed 3, Philadelphia, 1999, WB Saunders.

Halperin ML, Kamel KS: Potassium, *Lancet* 352(9122):135-140, 1998.

Halterman RK, Berl T: Therapy of dystremic disorders. In Brady HR, Wilcox CS, editors: *Therapy in nephrology and hypertension,* Philadelphia, 1999, WB Saunders.

Harding D, Cairns P, Gupta S et al: Hypernatremia: why bother weighing breast fed babies? *Arch Dis Child Fetal* 85(2): F145, 2001.

Hicks W, Hardy G: Phosphate supplementation for hypophosphataemia and parenteral nutrition, *Curr Opin Clin Nutr Metab Care* 4(3):227-233, 2001.

Hilton G: Emergency. Thermal burns, *AJN* 101(11):32-34, 2001.

Ho AM, Karmakar MK, Contardi LH et al: Excessive use of normal saline in managing traumatized patients in shock: a preventable contributor to acidosis, *J Trauma* 51(1):173-177, 2001.

Horne M: Endocrinologic dysfunctions. In Swearingen PL, Keen JH, editors: *Manual of critical care nursing: nursing interventions and collaborative management,* ed 4, St Louis, 2001, Mosby.

Johnson J: Burns. In Swearingen PL, Keen JH, editors: *Manual of critical care nursing: nursing interventions and collaborative management,* ed 4, St Louis, 2001, Mosby.

Jordan KS: Fluid resuscitation in acutely injured patients, *J Intraven Nurs* 23(2):81-87, 2000.

Kamel KS, Halperin ML: Treatment of hypokalemia and hyperkalemia. In Brady HR, Wilcox CS, editors: *Therapy in nephrology and hypertension,* Philadelphia, 1999, WB Saunders.

Kaplow R, Barry R: Continuous renal replacement therapy, *AJN* 120(11):26-34, 2002.

Krau SD: Selecting and managing fluid therapies. Colloids versus crystalloids, *Crit Care Nurs Clin North Am* 10(4):401-410, 1998.

Kenney WL, Chiu P: Influence of age on thirst and fluid intake, *Med Sci Sports Exerc* 33(9):1524-1532, 2001.

Khanna A, Kurtzman NA: Metabolic alkalosis, *Respir Care* 46(4): 354-365, 2001.

Kim MJ, McFarland GK, McLane AM: *Pocket guide to nursing diagnoses,* ed 7, St Louis, 1997, Mosby.

Kinney MR, Dunbar S, Brooks-Brunn JA et al: *AACN's clinical reference for critical care nursing,* ed 4, St Louis, 1998, Mosby.

Kirksey KM, Holt-Ashley M, Goodroad BK: An easy method for interpreting the results of arterial blood gas analysis, *Crit Care Nurse* 21(5):49-54, 2001.

Klein S, Kinney J, Jeejeebhoy K et al: Nutrition support in clinical practice: review of published data and recommendations for future research directions, *Am J Clin Nutr* 66(3):683-706, 1997.

Koko JP, Tannen RL, editors: *Fluids and electrolytes,* ed 3, Philadelphia, 1996, WB Saunders.

Koschel MJ: Where there's smoke, there may be cyanide, *AJN* 102(8):39-42, 2002.

Kraut JA, Madias NE: Approach to patients with acid base disorders, *Respir Care* 46(4):392-403, 2001.

Kumar S, Berl T: Sodium, *Lancet* 352(9123):220-228, 1998.

Laffey JG, Kavanagh BP: Hypocapnia, *N Engl J Med* 347(1):43-53, 2002.

Levin NW, Hoenich NA: Consequences of hyperphosphatemia and elevated levels of the calcium-phosphorus product in dialysis patients, *Curr Opin Nephrol Hypertens* 10(5):563-568, 2001.

Liao F, Folsom AR, Brancati FL: Is low magnesium concentration a risk factor for coronary disease? The Atherosclerosis Risk in Communities (ARIC) Study, *Am Heart J* 136(3):480-490, 1998.

Lowenstein J: *Acid and basics: a guide to understanding acid-base disorders,* New York, 1993, Oxford University.

Mandal AK: Hypokalemia and hyperkalemia, *Med Clin North Am* 81(3):611-639, 1997.

Marion BS: A turn for the better: prone positioning of patients with ARDS, *AJN* 101(5):26-34, 2001.

Matarese LE, Gottschlich MM, editors: *Contemporary nutrition support practice: a clinical guide,* Philadelphia, 1998, WB Saunders.

Mattu A, Brady WJ, Robinson DA: Electrocardiographic manifestations of hyperkalemia, *Am J Emerg Med* 18(6):721-729, 2000.

McCloskey JC, Bulechek GM, editors: *Nursing interventions classification (NIC),* ed 3, St Louis, 2000, Mosby.

Meininger ME, Kendler JS: Image in clinical medicine. Trousseau's sign, *N Engl J Med* 343(25):1855, 2000.

Miller-Catchpole R: Diagnostic and therapeutic technology assessment: transjugular intrahepatic portosystemic shunt (TIPS), *JAMA* 273(23):1824-1830, 1995.

Miller M: Hyponatremia: age related risk factors and therapy decisions, *Geriatrics* 53(7):32-42, 1998.

Milner SM, Mottar R, Smith CE: The Burn Wheel, *AJN* 101(11): 35-37, 2001.

Monk RD, Bushinsky DA: Treatment of calcium, phosphorus, and magnesium disorders. In Brady HR, Wilcox CS, editors: *Therapy in nephrology and hypertension,* Philadelphia, 1999, WB Saunders.

Moritz ML, Ayus JC: The changing pattern of hypernatremia in hospitalized children, *Pediatrics* 104(3 Pt 1):435-439, 1999.

Morrison RT: Edema and principles of diuretic use, *Med Clin North Am* 81(3):689-704, 1997.

Mundy GR, Guise TA: Hypercalcemia of malignancy, *Am J Med* 103(2):134-145, 1997.

Murray TA, Patterson LA: Prone positioning of trauma patients with acute respiratory distress syndrome and open abdominal incisions, *Crit Care Nurse* 22(3):52-56, 2002.

Narins RG, Emmett M: Simple and mixed acid-base disorders: a practical approach, *Medicine* 59(3):161-187, 1980.

National Osteoporosis Foundation: *Clinical updates,* 3(2):1-7, 2002.

North American Menopause Society: The role of calcium in peri- and postmenopausal women: consensus opinion of the North American Menopause Society, *Menopause* 8(2):84-95, 2001.

Oster JR, Singer I: Hyponatremia, hyposomolality, and hypotonicity: tables and fables, *Arch Intern Med* 159(4):333-336, 1999.

Osborn K: Nursing burn injuries, *Nurs Manage* 34(5):49-56, 2003.

Palevsky PM: Hypernatremia, *Semin Nephrol* 18(1):20-30, 1998.

Palevsky PM, Bhagrath R, Greenberg A: Hypernatremia in hospitalized patients, *Ann Intern Med* 124(2):197-203, 1996.

Parrillo J, Dellinger R, editors: *Critical care medicine: principles of diagnoses and management in the adult,* ed 2, Philadelphia, 2001, WB Saunders.

Perazella MA, Mahnensmith RL: Hyperkalemia in the elderly: drugs exacerbate impaired potassium homeostasis, *J Gen Intern Med* 12(10):646-656, 1997.

Pflederer TA: Emergency fluid management for hypovolemia, *Postgrad Med* 100(3):243-254, 1996.

Phipps WJ, Monahan FD, Sands JK et al: *Medical-surgical nursing: health and illness perspectives,* ed 7, St Louis, 2003, Mosby.

Preston RA: *Acid-base, fluids, and electrolytes—made ridiculously simple,* Miami, 1997, Med Master.

Rasool A, Palevsky PM: Treatment of edematous disorders with diuretics, *Am J Med Sci* 319(1):25-37, 2000.

Rastegar A, Soleimani M: Hypokalaemia and hyperkalaemia, *Postgrad Med J* 77(914):759-764, 2001.

Razavi B: Baking soda toxicity, *Am J Med* 108(9):756-757, 2000.

Rochon PA, Gill SS, Litner J et al: A systematic review of the evidence for hypodermoclysis to treat dehydration in older people, *J Gerontol A Biol Sci Med Sci* 52(3):M169-M176, 1997.

Rose BD: *Clinical physiology of acid-base and electrolyte disorders,* ed 5, New York, 2000, McGraw-Hill.

Rosenthal MH: Intraoperative fluid management: what and how much? *Chest* 115(suppl 5):106S-112S, 1999.

Schwetz BA: Hypercalcemia of malignancy, *JAMA* 286(13):1569, 2001.

See AC, Soo KC: Hypocalcemia following thyroidectomy for thyrotoxicosis, *Brit J Surg* 84(1):95-97, 1997.

Sheridan RL: Burns, *Crit Care Med* 30(suppl 11):S500-S514, 2002.

Shoulders-Odom B: Using an algorithm to interpret arterial blood gases, *Dimens Crit Care Nurs* 19(1):36-41, 2000.

Stern SA: Low-volume fluid resuscitation for presumed hemorrhagic shock: helpful or harmful? *Curr Opin Crit Care* 7(6):422-430, 2001.

Subramanian R, Khardori R: Severe hypophosphatemia: pathophysiologic implications, clinical presentations, and treatment, *Medicine* 79(1):1-8, 2000.

Swenson ER: Metabolic acidosis, *Resp Care* 46(4):342-353, 2001.

Thillainayagam AV, Hunt JB, Farthing MJ: Enhancing clinical efficacy of oral rehydration therapy: is low osmolality the key? *Gastroenterology* 114(1):197-210, 1998.

Toto KH: Fluid balance assessment: the total perspective, *Crit Care Nurs Clin North Am* 10(4):383-400, 1998.

Uhlig K, Sarnak MJ, Singh AK: New approaches to the treatment of calcium and phosphorus abnormalities in patients on hemodialysis, *Curr Opin Nephrol Hypertens* 10(6):793-798, 2001.

Van Amerongen RH, Moretta AC, Gaeta TJ: Severe hypernatremic dehydration and death in a breast-fed infant, *Pediatr Emerg Care* 17(3):175-180, 2001.

Vetter T, Lohse MJ: Magnesium and the parathyroid, *Curr Opin Nephrol Hypertens* 11(4):403-410, 2002.

Weigel RJ: Nonoperative management of hyperparathyroidism: present and future, *Curr Opin Oncol* 13(1):33-38, 2001.

Weiskittel P: Renal-urinary dysfunctions. In Swearingen PL, Keen JH, editors: *Manual of critical care nursing: nursing interventions and collaborative management,* ed 4, St Louis, 2001, Mosby.

# Appendix A

*Standard Abbreviations*

**ABA:** American Burn Association
**ABG:** Arterial blood gas
**ACE:** Angiotensin-converting enzyme
**ACTH:** Adrenocorticotropic hormone
**ADH:** Antidiuretic hormone
**AG:** Anion gap
**AIDS:** Acquired immunodeficiency syndrome
**ALS:** Amyotrophic lateral sclerosis
**ARB:** Angiotensin-receptor blocker
**ARDS:** Adult respiratory distress syndrome
**ARF:** Acute renal failure
**ATN:** Acute tubular necrosis
**ATP:** Adenosine triphosphate
**ATPase:** Adenosine triphosphatase
**AV:** Atrioventricular

**BEE:** Basal energy expenditure
**bid:** Two times a day
**BMI:** Body mass index
**BNP:** B-type natriuretic peptide
**BP:** Blood pressure
**bpm:** Beats per minute
**BSA:** Body surface area
**BUN:** Blood urea nitrogen

**C:** Celsius
**$Ca^{2+}$:** Calcium ion
**CAVH:** Continuous arteriovenous hemofiltration
**CBC:** Complete blood cell count
**CHF:** Congestive heart failure
**$Cl^-$:** Chloride ion

**cm:**   Centimeter
**cm $H_2O$:**   Centimeters of water
**CNS:**   Central nervous system
**CO:**   Cardiac output
**$CO_2$:**   Carbon dioxide
**COPD:**   Chronic obstructive pulmonary disease
**CPR:**   Cardiopulmonary resuscitation
**CRF:**   Chronic renal failure
**CVA:**   Cerebrovascular accident
**CVC:**   Central venous catheter
**CVP:**   Central venous pressure

**DDAVP:**   1-Deamino-8-D-arginine vasopressin
**DI:**   Diabetes insipidus
**DKA:**   Diabetic ketoacidosis
**dL:**   Deciliter
**DM:**   Diabetes mellitus
**DPG:**   Diphosphoglycerate
**$D_5W$:**   5% dextrose in water

**ECF:**   Extracellular fluid
**ECG:**   Electrocardiogram
**ECV:**   Effective circulating volume
**ESRD:**   End-stage renal disease

**F:**   Fahrenheit
**$Fio_2$:**   Fraction of inspired oxygen
**fl:**   Femtoliter

**g:**   Gram
**GFR:**   Glomerular filtration rate
**GI:**   Gastrointestinal

**$H^+$:**   Hydrogen ion
**$H_2CO_3$:**   Carbonic acid
**HCl:**   Hydrochloric acid
**$HCO_3^-$:**   Bicarbonate ion
**Hgb:**   Hemoglobin
**HHNK:**   Hyperosmolar hyperglycemic nonketotic
**HHNS:**   Hyperosmolar hyperglycemic nonketotic syndrome
**$HPO_4^{2-}$:**   Phosphate ion (*also abbreviated* $PO_4^{3-}$)
**HR:**   Heart rate

**ICF:**  Intracellular fluid
**ICP:**  Intracranial pressure
**IM:**  Intramuscular
**in:**  Inches
**I&O:**  Intake and output
**ISF:**  Interstitial fluid
**IU:**  International unit
**Iμ U:**  International microunit
**IV:**  Intravenous
**IVF:**  Intravascular fluid
**IVS:**  Intravascular space

**K$^+$:**  Potassium ion
**KCl:**  Potassium chloride
**kg:**  Kilogram

**L:**  Liter
**lb:**  Pound
**LCT:**  Long-chain triglyceride
**LOC:**  Level of consciousness

**m:**  Meter
**MAO:**  Monoamine oxidase
**MAP:**  Mean arterial pressure
**MCT:**  Medium-chain triglyceride
**mEq:**  Milliequivalent
**mg:**  Milligram
**Mg$^{2+}$:**  Magnesium ion
**MgSO$_4$:**  Magnesium sulfate
**MI:**  Myocardial infarction
**mL:**  Milliliter
**mm Hg:**  Millimeters of mercury
**mmol:**  Millimole
**mOsm:**  Milliosmole

**Na$^+$:**  Sodium ion
**NaCl:**  Sodium chloride
**NaHCO$_3$:**  Sodium bicarbonate
**ng:**  Nanogram
**NG:**  Nasogastric
**NH$_3$:**  Ammonia

**NH$_4^+$:**   Ammonium ion
**NPO:**   Nothing by mouth
**NS:**   Normal saline (i.e., isotonic solution of NaCl)
**NSAID:**   Nonsteroidal antiinflammatory drug

**O$_2$:**   Oxygen
**OG:**   Orogastric
**OTC:**   Over-the-counter
**oz:**   Ounce

**P:**   Phosphorus
**PA:**   Pulmonary artery
**Pa$_{CO_2}$:**   Partial pressure of carbon dioxide in arterial blood
**Pa$_{O_2}$:**   Partial pressure of oxygen in arterial blood
**PADP:**   Pulmonary artery diastolic pressure
**PAP:**   Pulmonary artery pressure
**PAWP:**   Pulmonary artery wedge pressure
**pg:**   Picogram
**PN:**   Parenteral nutrition
**PO:**   By mouth
**PO$_4^{3-}$:**   Phosphate ion (*also abbreviated* HPO$_4^{2-}$)
**PRBCs:**   Packed red blood cells
**prn:**   As needed
**PTH:**   Parathyroid hormone
**PVC:**   Premature ventricular contractions *or* peripheral venous catheter

**q:**   Every
**qd:**   Every day

**RBC:**   Red blood cell
**RDA:**   Recommended daily allowance
**ROM:**   Range of motion
**RR:**   Respiratory rate
**RTA:**   Renal tubular acidosis

**SC:**   Subcutaneous
**SIADH:**   Syndrome of inappropriate secretion of antidiuretic hormone
**SOB:**   Shortness of breath
**stat:**   Immediately

**SVR:**   Systemic vascular resistance

**TBSA:**   Total body surface area
**TBW:**   Total body water
**TCF:**   Transcellular fluid
**tid:**   Three times a day
**TIPS:**   Transjugular intrahepatic portosystemic shunt
**TNA:**   Total nutrient admixture
**TPN:**   Total parenteral nutrition
**TSF:**   Triceps skinfold

**U:**   Unit
**μg:**   Microgram
**μ IU:**   Microinternational unit
**μm:**   Micrometer

**VS:**   Vital signs

**WBC:**   White blood cell
**WOB:**   Work of breathing

# Appendix B

*Glossary*

**Acidemia:**  Change of pH in arterial blood to less than 7.40.

**Acidosis:**  Abnormal accumulation of acid or loss of base from the body.

**Acids:**  Substances that can give up a hydrogen ion.

**Active transport:**  The movement of solutes across a cell membrane in the absence of a favorable electrochemical or concentration gradient; requires energy.

**Acute renal failure (ARF):**  A sudden loss of renal function that is usually reversible.

**Aldosterone:**  A mineralocorticoid hormone released by the adrenal cortex that increases the resorption (saving) of sodium and the secretion and excretion of potassium and hydrogen by the kidneys.

**Alkalemia:**  Increase in arterial pH to more than 7.40.

**Alkalosis:**  Abnormal accumulation of bicarbonate or loss of acid in the body.

**Anaerobic metabolism:**  Occurs when not enough oxygen is available for metabolism and alternate pathways are used, resulting in an accumulation of organic acids (lactic acidosis).

**Analog:**  A substance with structure and function similar to another substance.

**Anasarca:**  Severe generalized edema.

**Angiotensin:**  A polypeptide found in the blood and formed by the action of renin on the $\alpha$-2-globulin angiotensinogen. *Angiotensin I* is converted to *angiotensin II*. Angiotensin II, a potent vasoconstrictor, acts on the adrenal cortex to stimulate the release of aldosterone.

**Anions:**  Ions that develop a negative charge in solution. Examples of the body's most common anions include chloride ion, bicarbonate ion, and phosphate ion. Proteins are another important group of anions.

**Anion gap:** Reflection of the anions in plasma (e.g., phosphates, sulfates, proteinates) that normally are unmeasured. Anion gap is helpful in the differential diagnosis of metabolic acidosis or mixed acid-base disorders.

**Antidiuretic hormone (ADH):** Produced by the hypothalamus and released by the posterior pituitary gland, it increases resorption (saving) of water by the kidneys, allowing excretion of a concentrated urine. In addition, ADH is an arterial vasoconstrictor that increases blood pressure by increasing vascular resistance.

**Anuria:** The production of less than 100 mL of urine in 24 hours.

**Arterial blood gases (ABGs):** Measurement of pH, carbon dioxide tension, and oxygen tension of arterial blood to evaluate acid-base and pulmonary functions.

**Asterixis:** Hand-flapping tremor that occurs with extension of the arm and dorsiflexion of the wrist. It is often seen with metabolic disorders.

**Azotemia:** Increased retention of metabolic wastes.

**Baroreceptors:** Pressure-sensitive nerve endings located in the carotid sinuses, aortic arch, cardiac atria, and renal vessels that respond to changes in blood pressure via changes in stretch in the arterial wall, leading to changes in cardiac output, vascular resistance, thirst, and renal handling of sodium and water.

**Bases:** Substances that can take on a hydrogen ion.

**Bicarbonate ($HCO_3^-$):** The body's most important and abundant buffer. It is generated in the kidney and aids in excretion of hydrogen ion.

**B-type natriuretic peptide:** Natriuretic peptide produced by the ventricular myocardium. See natriuretic peptides.

**Buffers:** Substances that combine with excess acid or base, resulting in a minimally altered pH.

**Capillary membrane:** Separates the intravascular fluid from the interstitial fluid.

**Cardiac output (CO):** Product of heart rate × stroke volume (i.e., the amount of blood moved with each contraction of the left ventricle per minute). Normal value is 4 to 7 L/minute for the adult.

**Catabolic:**   Breaking down in the body of complex substances into simpler ones, usually accompanied by the release of energy. Catabolic state usually refers to the breakdown of tissue.

**Cations:**   Ions that develop a positive charge in solution and are attracted to negative electrons. Examples of the body's most common cations include sodium ions, potassium ions, calcium ions, magnesium ions, and hydrogen ions.

**Cell membrane:**   Composed of lipids and protein, this membrane separates intracellular fluid from interstitial fluid.

**Central venous pressure (CVP):**   Measurement of the right atrial pressure and right ventricular end-diastolic pressure via a catheter inserted in or near the right atrium.

**Chronic renal failure (CRF):**   An irreversible loss of kidney function, also known as *end-stage renal disease (ESRD)*.

**Chvostek's sign:**   A signal of tetany occurring with hypocalcemia or hypomagnesemia; considered positive when there is unilateral contraction of the facial and eyelid muscles in response to facial nerve percussion.

**Colloid:**   In the medical vernacular, colloid is an intravenous fluid that contains solutes that do not readily cross the capillary membrane. Dextran, blood, albumin, mannitol, and plasma are all colloids. When combined with water, colloids do not form true solutions.

**Concentration gradient:**   The concentration difference between an area of a high concentration and an area of low concentration in the same substance.

**Crystalloid:**   In the medical vernacular, crystalloid is an intravenous fluid that contains solutes that readily cross the capillary membrane. Examples include dextrose or electrolyte solutions. When combined with water, crystalloids dissolve and form true solutions.

**Diffusion:**   Random movement of particles through a solution or gas in which the particles move from an area of high concentration to an area of low concentration. When diffusion of a particular solute is dependent on the availability of a carrier substance, it is termed *facilitated* *diffusion*. Diffusion not dependent on a carrier substance is termed *simple diffusion*.

**Edema:** Palpable swelling of the interstitial space that can be either localized or generalized.

**Effective circulating volume (ECV):** The portion of intravascular volume that actually perfuses the tissues. For example, in congestive heart failure, intravascular volume increases because of sodium and water retention, yet ECV decreases because of the pooling of blood in the venous circuit.

**Effective osmolality:** Changes in osmolality that cause water to move from one compartment to another. If a substance has an equal concentration on both sides of the membrane, there is no effective osmolality. *Tonicity* is another term for effective osmolality.

**Electrolytes:** Substances (solutes) that dissociate in solution and conduct an electric current. Electrolytes dissociate into positive ions (cations) and negative ions (anions).

**Epithelial membrane:** Separates interstitial fluid and intravascular fluid from the transcellular fluid; also produces transcellular fluid.

**Erythropoietin:** A glycoprotein hormone released by the renal cells in response to low oxygen levels that stimulates production of red blood cells by the bone marrow.

**Eschar:** A thick crust or slough that develops after a thermal burn.

**Extravasation:** Act of fluid escaping from a vessel into the tissue, most commonly referring to leakage from a blood vessel.

**Extracellular fluid (ECF):** Fluid found outside the cells, making up approximately one third of the body's fluid (in the adult).

**Filtration:** Movement of water and solutes from an area of high hydrostatic pressure to an area of low hydrostatic pressure.

**Glomerular filtration rate (GFR):** The volume of fluid crossing the glomerular membrane each minute.

**Hemolysis:**  Breakdown of red blood cells that may occur if blood is exposed to a hypotonic solution.

**Homeostasis:**  Physiologic balance in which there is relative constancy in the body's environment; maintained by adaptive responses.

**Hydraulic pressure:**  One of the factors that affects the movement of fluid across the capillary membrane. It is a combination of hydrostatic pressure and the pressure created by the pump action of the heart. The terms *hydrostatic pressure* and *hydraulic pressure* are often used interchangeably.

**Hydrostatic pressure:**  Pressure created by the weight of fluid.

**Hypercapnia:**  Increased amounts of carbon dioxide in the blood caused by hypoventilation; also known as *hypercarbia.*

**Hypertonicity:**  State in which a solution's effective osmolality is greater than that of the body's fluids.

**Hyperventilation:**  Any process resulting in a decreased $Paco_2$.

**Hypervolemia:**  Expansion of the extracellular fluid volume. Usually used to describe the expansion of the intravascular portion of the extracellular fluid.

**Hypocapnia:**  Decreased amounts of carbon dioxide in the blood caused by hyperventilation; also known as *hypocarbia.*

**Hypotonicity:**  State in which a solution's effective osmolality is less than that of the body's fluids.

**Hypoventilation:**  Any process resulting in an increased $Paco_2$.

**Hypovolemia:**  Reduction in the extracellular fluid volume. Usually used to describe a reduction in the volume of the intravascular portion of the extracellular fluid.

**Insensible fluid:**  Imperceptible loss of fluid through the skin or respiratory system via evaporation. Because it is nearly free of electrolytes, insensible fluid loss is considered pure water loss.

**Interstitial fluid (ISF):**  The fluid surrounding the cells, including lymph fluid.

**Intracellular fluid (ICF):**  Fluid contained within the cells, making up approximately two thirds of the body's fluid (in the adult).

**Intravascular fluid (IVF):**   Fluid contained within the blood vessels (e.g., plasma).

**Isohydric principle:**   Principle stating that a change in the hydrogen ion concentration affects the ratio of acids to bases in all buffer systems.

**Isotonic solutions:**   Fluids with the same effective osmolality as body fluids.

**Kussmaul's respirations:**   Rapid, deep, sighing breaths.

**Mean arterial pressure (MAP):**   A reflection of the average pressure within the arterial tree throughout the cardiac cycle. The normal value is 70 to 105 mm Hg.

**Metastatic calcifications:**   Precipitation and deposition of calcium phosphate in the soft tissue, joints, and arteries; also known as *soft tissue calcifications.*

**Milk-alkali syndrome:**   Renal dysfunction and metabolic alkalosis resulting from chronic ingestion of excessive amounts of absorbable alkali (e.g., milk and calcium carbonate).

**Minute ventilation:**   Respiratory rate × tidal volume.

**Natriuretic peptides:**   Family of peptide hormones affecting fluid volume status and cardiovascular function through increased excretion of sodium (natriuresis), direct vasodilation, and opposition of the renin-angiotensin-aldosterone system.

**Nonelectrolytes:**   Substances that do not dissociate (separate) in solution (e.g., glucose, urea, creatinine, bilirubin).

**Nonvolatile (fixed) acid:**   Any acid that cannot be vaporized and excreted by the lungs.

**Oliguria:**   Urinary output of less than 400 mL in 24 hours.

**Oncotic pressure:**   Osmotic pressure exerted by protein.

**Osmolality:**   Osmotic concentration of body fluids (i.e., the number of dissolved substances per kilogram of water); measured in mOsm/kg of water.

**Osmolarity:**   Like osmolality, *osmolarity* is a term used to describe the concentration of fluids; measured in mOsm/L of solution.

**Osmosis:**   Movement of water across a semipermeable membrane from an area of lower solute concentration to an area of higher solute concentration.

**Osmotic diuresis:** Increased urine output caused by such substances as mannitol, glucose, or contrast media, which are excreted in the urine and reduce water resorption.

**Osmotic pressure:** The pressure that pulls water across a semipermeable membrane when the membrane separates two solutions with different concentrations.

**Oxygen saturation:** The degree to which hemoglobin is combined with oxygen.

**pH:** Measurement of hydrogen ion concentration in body fluids reflecting one of the following states: normal (7.40), acidic ( < 7.40), or alkalotic ( > 7.40).

**Plasma:** The fluid portion of the blood, containing water, protein, and electrolytes.

**Polyuria:** Excessive urine output.

**Pulmonary artery pressure (PAP):** Pressure measured in the pulmonary artery. When pulmonary function is normal, it reflects the pressure within the left ventricle at the end of diastole. PAP is used to evaluate left ventricular function and fluid volume. Normal PAP is 20 to 30/8 to 15 mm Hg.

**Pulmonary artery wedge pressure (PAWP):** Measurement of pulmonary capillary pressure with a balloon-tipped catheter passed into the distal pulmonary artery. It provides a more accurate reflection of left ventricular end-diastolic pressure than pulmonary artery pressure. Normal PAWP is 6 to 12 mm Hg.

**Renin:** Proteolytic enzyme produced and released by specialized cells located in the arterioles of the kidney. Renin is released in response to decreased renal perfusion or stimulation of the sympathetic nervous system and is important in the formation of angiotensin.

**Sensible fluid:** Perceptible loss of body fluid (e.g., sweat) via the skin; contains a significant amount of electrolytes.

**Serum:** Plasma, minus the fibrinogen and other clotting factors (i.e., the fluid that remains after a blood specimen has been allowed to form a clot).

**Sodium-potassium pump:** A physiologic mechanism present in all body cell membranes that transports sodium from the inside of the cell to the outside and transports potassium from the outside of the cell to the inside; requires energy and the presence of adequate magnesium.

**Solutes:** Dissolved particles found in body fluids. There are two types: electrolytes and nonelectrolytes.

**Specific gravity:** Measurement of the weight of a substance in relationship to water; water = 1.000.

**Substrate:** A substance that is acted on (and changed by) an enzyme during a chemical reaction.

**Syndrome of inappropriate secretion of antidiuretic hormone (SIADH):** A condition in which there is inappropriate hypothalamic production or enhanced action or ectopic production of antidiuretic hormone, resulting in excess water retention.

**Systemic vascular resistance (SVR):** Clinical measurement of the resistance in vessels, which is used to determine workload of the left ventricle (afterload). Normal SVR is 900 to 1200 dynes/second/cm$^{-5}$.

**Tachypnea:** Increased respiratory rate; also called *hyperpnea*.

**Third-space fluid shift:** The loss of extracellular fluid into a normally nonequilibrating space. Although the fluid has not been lost from the body, it is temporarily unavailable to the intracellular fluid or extracellular fluid for its use.

**Tidal volume:** Normal resting volume of ventilation.

**Tonicity:** Another term for effective osmolality.

**Transcellular fluid (TCF):** Fluid secreted by epithelial cells. These fluids include cerebrospinal, pericardial, pleural, synovial, and intraocular fluids and digestive secretions.

**Trousseau's sign:** Ischemia-induced carpal spasm that occurs with hypocalcemia and hypomagnesemia; may be elicited by applying a blood pressure cuff to the upper arm and inflating it past systolic blood pressure for 2 minutes.

**Ventilation-perfusion mismatch:** An inequality in the ratio between ventilation and perfusion that occurs with shunting of venous blood past unventilated alveoli.

**Volatile acid:** An acid that can be vaporized and eliminated by the lungs (e.g., carbon dioxide).

# Appendix C

*Effects of Age on Fluid, Electrolyte, and Acid-Base Balance*

## Infants and Children

- Relative to their size, infants and children have a greater body surface area (BSA; both external and internal) than adults and thus have a greater potential for fluid loss via the skin and gastrointestinal (GI) tract.
- Infants and children have a higher percentage of total body water (TBW) than adults. The greater percentage of the infant's body water is extracellular. As cellular growth occurs, more fluid becomes intracellular.
- Infants have a decreased ability to concentrate their urine; at the same time, they have an increased solute load to excrete because of their increased caloric need. These two factors result in a relatively greater obligatory fluid loss, meaning that they must produce a relatively larger volume of urine to excrete their daily load of metabolic wastes.
- The daily intake and output (I&O) for infants (e.g., 650 mL) is equal to approximately half the volume of their extracellular fluid (ECF; e.g., 1300 mL), as compared with adults whose daily I&O (e.g., 2500 mL) is approximately one sixth of their ECF (e.g., 15 L). Thus infants can lose a volume equal to their ECF in 2 days, and it takes an adult 6 days.
- Because of an infant's small size and decreased ability to excrete excess fluid, intravenous (IV) fluid administration necessitates caution (e.g., use of monitored pumps).
- Infants are less able to compensate for acidosis because of their decreased ability to acidify urine.
- Infants are at increased risk for development of hypernatremia because they are unable to verbalize feelings of thirst.

Thirst is the body's primary defense against symptomatic hypernatremia.

- Children have an increased incidence and intensity of fever, upper respiratory infections, and gastroenteritis, which can lead to abnormal fluid and electrolyte loss. Diarrhea is the most common cause of fluid and electrolyte imbalance. (See Chapter 18 for a discussion of various fluid and electrolyte imbalances that occur with loss of upper and lower GI contents.)

- Young children are at greater risk for hypokalemia because their kidneys excrete potassium in the face of decreased or absent potassium intake.

- Infants and small children are prone to fluid volume deficit caused by a combination of the factors listed previously. Unfortunately, some of the common indicators of fluid volume deficit are less reliable in the infant or small child. Infants are unable to verbalize feelings of thirst, although their cries may become increasingly high-pitched. Skin turgor also may be a less reliable sign. Skin turgor may appear normal in an obese infant because of increased subcutaneous (SC) fat, or it may appear abnormal in an adequately hydrated but undernourished infant. Irritability is an early indicator of hypovolemia. Sunken fontanels, a traditional indicator of dehydration, do not occur until there has been moderate to severe fluid loss.

## Older Adults

- Weight (body fat) tends to increase with advancing age; thus the percentage of TBW decreases. (Fat cells contain little water.) The percentage of TBW increases in an emaciated individual who has lost significant body fat.

- Renal function decreases with advancing age. Glomerular filtration rate (GFR) drops; thus an older adult is less likely to compensate for an increased metabolic load. There is also a reduction in the ability to concentrate urine, resulting in greater obligatory water losses. An older adult must produce a larger volume of urine to excrete the same amount of metabolic waste as a younger adult.

- In older adults, the kidneys are less able to compensate for an acid load, resulting in decreased ammonia formation.

(Ammonia produced by the renal tubular cell diffuses into the lumen of the tubule and combines with hydrogen to form ammonium, which is then excreted in the urine. In this way, ammonia acts as a urinary buffer, allowing increased excretion of hydrogen ions.) Normally, ammonia production increases in the presence of an acid load.

- Decreased respiratory function reduces an older adult's ability to compensate for acid-base imbalance. Maximum respiratory compensation for metabolic acidosis can decrease the $Paco_2$ to 20 mm Hg in older adults, and the $Paco_2$ can drop to 10 to 15 mm Hg in a younger person. An older adult is also more likely to have hypoxemia develop.
- There is a reduction in the secretion of hydrochloric acid (HCl) by the stomach, which may affect an individual's ability to tolerate certain foods. Older adults are especially prone to constipation because of decreased GI tract motility. Limited fluid intake, a restricted diet, and a reduced level of physical activity may contribute to the development of constipation. Excessive or inappropriate use of laxatives may lead to problems with diarrhea.
- As the skin ages, there is a reduction in insensible and sensible water loss as a result of decreased skin hydration and decreased functioning of the sweat glands. Thus the skin is less efficient in cooling the body and the skin tends to be dry. In addition, skin turgor is a less reliable indicator of fluid status as a result of decreased skin elasticity.
- Older adults are at increased risk for development of hypernatremia because they have a less sensitive thirst center and may have problems with obtaining fluids (e.g., impaired mobility) or expressing their desire for fluids (e.g., an individual with expressive aphasia). Thirst is the body's primary defense against symptomatic hypernatremia.
- Older adults may have less tachycardia and a greater fall in blood pressure with hypovolemia from autonomic insufficiency.

# Appendix D

*Normal Laboratory Values and
New Blood Pressure Guidelines**

| Complete Blood Cell Count | Adult Normal Values |
|---|---|
| Hemoglobin | Male: 14-18 g/dL |
| | Female: 12-16 g/dL |
| Hematocrit | Male: 40%-54% |
| | Female: 37%-47% |
| Red blood cell count | Male: 4.5-6 million/$\mu$L |
| | Female: 4-5.5 million/$\mu$L |
| White blood cell count | 4500-11,000/$\mu$L |
|   Neutrophils | 54%-75% (3000-7500/$\mu$L) |
|   Band neutrophils | 3%-8% (150-700/$\mu$L) |
|   Lymphocytes | 25%-40% (1500-4500/$\mu$L) |
|   Monocytes | 2%-8% (100-500/$\mu$L) |
|   Eosinophils | 1%-4% (50-400/$\mu$L) |
|   Basophils | 0%-1% (25-100/$\mu$L) |
| Platelet count | 150,000-400,000/$\mu$L |

*Normal values may vary significantly with different laboratory methods of
testing.

| Serum, Plasma, and Whole Blood Chemistry | Normal Values |
| --- | --- |
| ACTH | 8 AM-10 AM: < 100 pg/mL |
| ADH | 0-2 pg/mL/serum osmolality < 285 mOsm/kg; 2-12 pg/mL/serum osmolality; > 290 mOsm/kg |
| Albumin | 3.5-5.5 g/dL |
| Aldosterone | Male: 6-22 ng/dL |
| | Female: 4-31 ng/dL |
| Ammonia | Adult: 15-110 µg/dL |
| | Child: 56-80 µg/dL |
| | Newborn: 90-150 µg/dL |
| Amylase | 60-180 Somogyi U/dL |
| Base, total | 145-160 mEq/L |
| Bicarbonate | 22-26 mmol/L |
| Bilirubin | Total: 0.3-1.4 mg/dL |
| ABGs | |
| pH | 7.35-7.45 |
| $Paco_2$ | 35-45 mm Hg |
| $Pao_2$ | 80-95 mm Hg |
| $O_2$ saturation | 95%-99% |
| Blood urea nitrogen | 6-20 mg/dL |
| Calcitonin | < 100 pg/mL |
| Calcium, total | 8.5-10.5 mg/dL; 4.3-5.3 mEq/L |
| Calcium, ionized | 4.5-5.1 mg/dL |
| Chloride | 95-108 mmol/L |
| Cortisol | 8 AM-10 AM: 5-25 µg/dL |
| | 4 PM-12 AM (midnight): 2-18 µg/dL |
| $CO_2$ content (total $CO_2$) | 22-28 mmol/L |
| CPK | Male: 55-170 U/L |
| | Female: 30-135 U/L |
| Creatinine | 0.6-1.5 mg/dL |
| Creatinine clearance | Male: 107-141 mL/minute |
| | Female: 87-132 mL/minute |

*ABGs,* Arterial blood gases; *ACTH,* adrenocorticotropic hormone; *ADH,* antidiuretic hormone; *$CO_2$,* carbon dioxide; *CPK,* creatinine phosphokinase; *$O_2$,* oxygen; *$Paco_2$,* partial pressure of carbon dioxide in arterial blood; *$Pao_2$,* partial pressure of oxygen in arterial blood.

| Serum, Plasma, and Whole Blood Chemistry | Normal Values |
| --- | --- |
| Globulins, total | 1.5-3.5 g/dL |
| Glucose, fasting | True glucose: 65-110 mg/dL |
| | All sugars: 80-120 mg/dL |
| Glucose, 2-hour postprandial | < 145 mg/dL |
| Glucose tolerance | |
| Intravenous | Fasting: 65-110 mg/dL |
| | 5-minute: maximum 250 mg/dL |
| | 60-minute: decrease |
| | 2-hour: < 120 mg/dL |
| | 3-hour: 65-110 mg/dL |
| Oral | Fasting: 65-110 mg/dL |
| | 30-minute: < 155 mg/dL |
| | 1-hour: < 165 mg/dL |
| | 2-hour: < 120 mg/dL |
| | 3-hour: ≤65-110 mg/dL |
| 17-OCHS | Male: 7-19 µg/dL |
| | Female: 9-21 µg/dL |
| Insulin | 11-240 µ IU/mL |
| | 4-24 µ U/mL |
| Iron | Total: 60-200 µg/dL |
| | Male, average: 125 µg/dL |
| | Female, average: 100 µg/dL |
| | Older adults: 60-80 µg/dL |
| Ketone bodies | 2-4 µg/dL |
| Lactic acid | Arterial: 0.5-1.6 mEq/L |
| | Venous: 1.5-2.2 mEq/L |
| Magnesium | 1.8-3 mg/dL |
| | 1.5-2.5 mEq/L |
| Osmolality | 280-300 mOsm/kg |
| Parathyroid hormone | < 2000 pg/mL |
| Phosphatase, acid | 0-1.1 U/mL (Bodansky) |
| | 1-4 U/mL (King-Armstrong) |
| | 0.13-0.63 U/mL (Bessey-Lowery) |

| Serum, Plasma, and Whole Blood Chemistry | Normal Values |
|---|---|
| Phosphatase, alkaline | 1.5-4.5 U/dL (Bodansky) |
| | 4-13 U/dL (King-Armstrong) |
| | 0.8-2.3 U/mL (Bessey-Lowery) |
| Phosphorus | 2.5-4.5 mg/dL; 0.81-1.45 mmol/L |
| Potassium | 3.5-5 mmol/L |
| Renin | Normal sodium intake |
| |   Supine (4-6 hours): |
| |   0.5-1.6 ng/mL/hour |
| |   Sitting (4 hours): |
| |   1.8-3.6 ng/mL/hour |
| | Low sodium intake |
| |   Supine (4-6 hours): |
| |   2.2-4.4 ng/mL/hour |
| |   Sitting (4 hours): |
| |   4-8.1 ng/mL/hour |
| Sodium | 135-145 mmol/L |
| Thyroid-stimulating hormone | 4.6 μ U/mL |
| Urea clearance | |
| Serum/24-hour urine | 64-99 mL/minute (maximum clearance) |
| Uric acid | 41-65 mL/minute (standard clearance) |
| | Male: 2.1-7.5 mg/dL |
| | Female: 2-6.6 mg/dL |

| Urine Chemistry | Normal Values |
|---|---|
| Albumin | |
| Random | Negative |
| 24-hour | 10-100 mg/24 hours |
| Amylase | |
| 2-hour | 35-260 (Somogyi) U/hour |
| 24-hour | 80-5000 U/24 hours |
| Bilirubin | |
| Random | Negative: 0.02 mg/dL |
| Calcium | |
| Random | 1 + turbidity; 10 mg/dL |
| 24-hour | 50-300 mg/24 hours |
| Creatinine | |
| 24-hour | Male: 20-26 mg/kg/24 hours |
| | Female: 14-22 mg/kg/24 hours |
| Creatinine clearance | Male: 107-141 mL/minute |
| | Female: 87-132 mL/minute |
| Glucose | |
| Random | Negative: 15 mg/dL |
| 24-hour | 130 mg/24 hours |
| Ketone | |
| 24-hour | Negative: 0.3-2 mg/dL |
| Osmolality | |
| Random | 350-700 mOsm/kg |
| 24-hour | 300-900 mOsm/kg |
| Physiologic range | 50-1200 mOsm/kg |
| pH | |
| Random | 4.6-8 |
| Phosphorus | |
| 24-hour | 0.9-1.3 g; 0.2-0.6 mEq/L |
| Protein | |
| Random | Negative: 2-8 mg/dL |
| 24-hour | 40-150 mg |

| Urine Chemistry | Normal Values |
|---|---|
| Sodium | |
| Random | 50-130 mmol/L |
| 24-hour | 40-220 mmol/L |
| Specific gravity | |
| Random | 1.010-1.020 |
| After fluid restriction | 1.025-1.035 |
| Sugar | |
| Random | Negative |
| Urea clearance | |
| 24-hour | 64-99 mL/minute (maximum) |
| | 41-65 mL/minute (standard) |
| Urea nitrogen | |
| 24-hour | 6-17 g |

## Classification of blood pressure

| Category | Systolic | | Diastolic |
|---|---|---|---|
| Normal | < 120 | and | < 80 |
| Prehypertension | 120-139 | or | 80-89 |
| Hypertension, stage 1 | 140-159 | or | 90-99 |
| Hypertension, stage 2 | ≥160 | or | ≥100 |

From Seventh Report of the Joint National Committee on Prevention,
Detection, Evaluation, and Treatment of High Blood Pressure, JNC 7,
May 2003, US Department of Health and Human Services,
National Institutes of Health; National Heart, Lung, and Blood Institute.

# Index

---

Page numbers followed by f indicate
figures; t, tables; b, boxes.